AF586926

GMP in Pharmaceutical Industry

Global cGMP & Regulatory Expectations

GMP in Pharmaceutical Industry

Global cGMP & Regulatory Expectations

Trupti Patil-Dongare

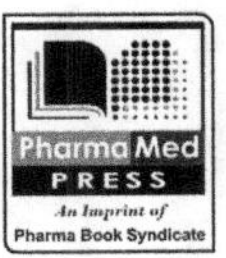

PharmaMed Press
An imprint of Pharma Book Syndicate
A unit of BSP Books Pvt. Ltd.
4-4-309/316, Giriraj Lane,
Sultan Bazar, Hyderabad - 500 095.

GMP in Pharmaceutical Industry: Global cGMP and Regulatory Expectations
by Trupti Patil-Dongare

Published by

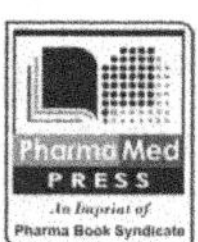

PharmaMed Press
An imprint of Pharma Book Syndicate
A unit of BSP Books Pvt. Ltd.
4-4-309/316, Giriraj Lane, Sultan Bazar, Hyderabad - 500 095.
Phone: 040-23445688, 23445600; Fax: 91+40-23445611
E-mail: info@pharmamedpress.com
www.pharmamedpress.com/pharmamedpress.net

ISBN: 978-93-88305-14-3 (Hardback)

FOREWORD

In the recent past, pharmaceutical manufacturing organizations worldwide have devoted a great deal of resources to ensure compliance with cGMP guidelines as issued by the licensing authorities. The Pharmaceutical industry, in particular, has demonstrated remarkably its ability to comply with the stringent requirements of regulatory authorities like the USFDA, European, MHRA and other regulatory bodies, a prerequisite to enter the lucrative generic market in the regulatory.

While many manufacturing units in India are already in compliance with the requirements of these stringent guidelines, a large number of medium and small-scale units still need to upgrade their facilities and procedures to comply with these requirements. Apart from facilities and systems involved in the manufacturer of pharmaceuticals, the current guideline lay great emphasis on the documentation of the procedures used to manufacture and store pharmaceutical products. This upgradation of the systems and procedures are essential to ensure a uniform quality product reducing the possibility of inter-batch and multiple locations.

In view of these changes, implemented by drug licensing authorities all over the world, I am happy these will be easily understood for greater benefit of the pharmaceutical industry, through this book. I am confident that this book will become a comprehensive reference guide for all technical personnel in the entire drug industry, especially personnel involved with the manufacturer of pharmaceutical formulation. More efforts such as these will go on long way in creating great awareness of these revised guidelines and will help to develop better preparedness among our technical personnel to face audits from different regulatory authorities in developed and developing countries.

- Sudhir Dongare

PREFACE

Drugs being a very important component of healthcare, these need special attention especially with respect to Quality, Efficacy and Safety. This has always been a matter of concern from the consumer point of view.

In India, initially drugs were imported. After Nineteen Hundred fifties, the Indian Pharmaceutical Industry has made phenomenal progress and reached the present state where now India exports both bulk drugs and formulations even to the developed countries as against a situation till Nineteen Hundred Forties when India was importing formulation.

Such growth and acceptance of products in the international market could happen only if Indian products could meet the quality standards as set by the International Regulator's.

The Quality Control concept is basically meant that the quality of the product conformed to pre-determined standards as given in the Pharmacopeia.

If the drugs are to qualify for export to non-regulatory market, then it can be only with assurance that products are manufactured as per the GMP guidelines defined in Schedule M or as per International regulatory guideline.

The pharmaceutical products must only be produced by licensed manufacturers, holders of the Manufacturing Authorization and whose activities are regularly inspected by the relevant National Sanitary Authorities. This Regulation of Good Manufacturing Practices (GMP) must be taken as a reference during the inspection of the plant facilities, of the production processes and quality control, and as training material for the inspectors in pharmaceutical products area, as well as, for the training of professionals responsible for the production process and Quality Control in the industries.

The GMP are applicable to all operations related to pharmaceutical products manufacturing, including those medicines being developed for clinical assays.

The Good Manufacturing Practices (GMP) described in this document are subject to continuous updating, keeping up with the evolution of new technologies, where alternative actions might be adapted to attend to necessities of a determined product, provided that alternative actions are validated to guarantee the product quality. The GMP do not contain aspects linked to the safety of the staff involved in the manufacturing process; those aspects are ruled by a specific legislation. Nevertheless, the manufacturer must guarantee the safety of his workers.

To compile this book Good Manufacturing Practices in Pharmaceutical Industry, a humble attempt has been made to bring the various GMP guidelines under one reference book.

It is sincerely hoped that the compilation of various cGMP guideline in this book in a simple language will help in bringing about harmonization of the quality systems in all big and small Pharma companies.

The implementation of cGMP and harmonized quality systems will ensure that there are no complaints and product recalls through continual improvement in Quality Systems which can be achieved through self-assessment. It will also ensure Active Pharmaceutical Ingredients and Formulations meeting standards of quality, efficacy and safety, thereby meeting customer satisfaction and the demand for export in International Markets.

- Trupti PatilDongare

CONTENTS

CHAPTER 18

Quality by Design (QbD) Approach in the Product Life Cycle

CHAPTER 19

Process Validation in Pharmaceutical Industry

CHAPTER 20

Cleaning Validation and Cross Contamination Approach on Risk MaPP Concept

CHAPTER 21

Pharmaceutical Water Generation and Distribution System and Regulatory Expectation

CHAPTER 22

Pharmaceutical Heating, Ventilation and Air Conditionings (HVAC) and Regulatory Expectations

CHAPTER 23

Manufacturing Execution System (MES) in Pharmaceutical Industry

CHAPTER 24

Pharmaceutical Drug Master File

CHAPTER 25

Common Technical Document in Regulatory Filing

CHAPTER 26

European Union Marketing Authorization

CHAPTER 27

Site Master File

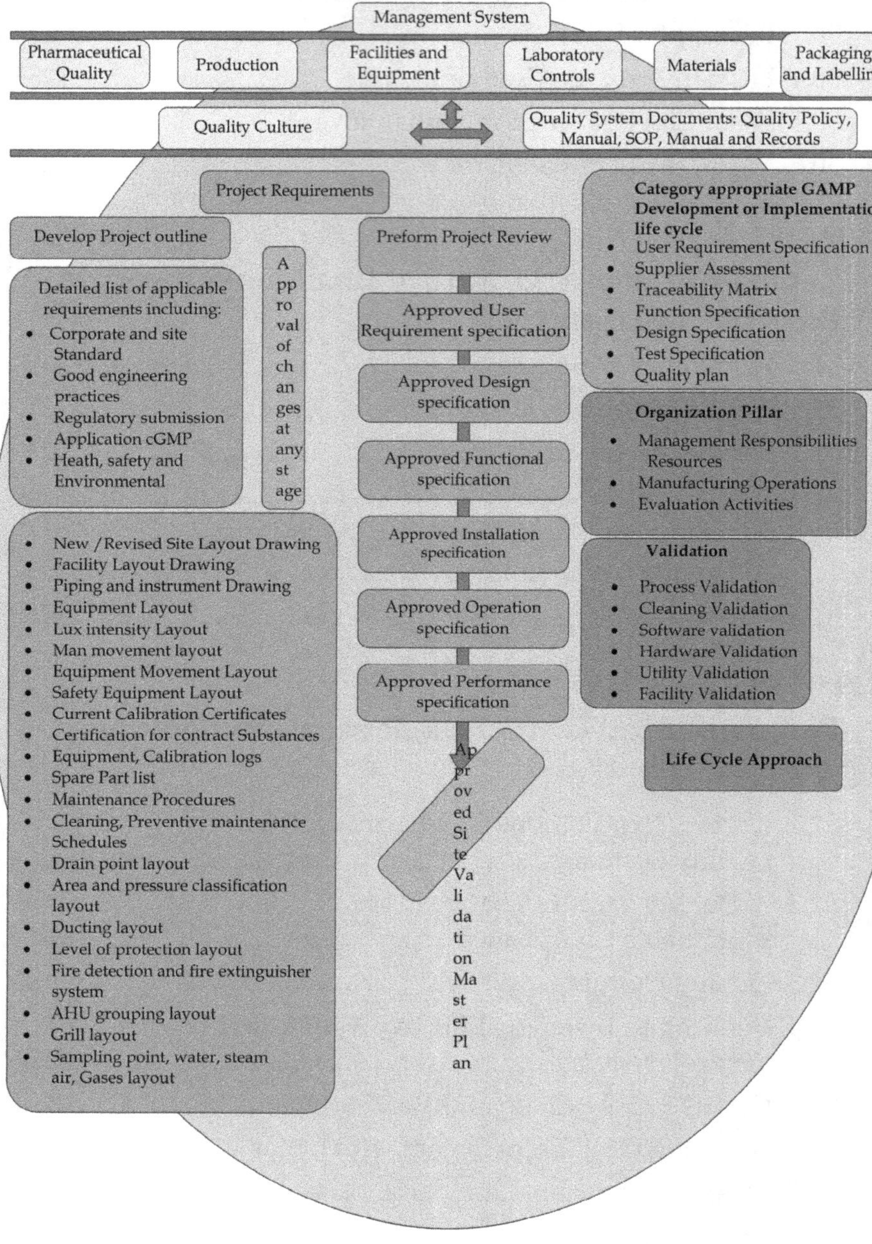
THE STANDARD ROUTE OF GMP
Management System
Pharmaceutical Quality
Production
Facilities and Equipment
Laboratory Controls
Materials
Packaging and Labelling
Quality Culture
Quality System Documents: Quality Policy, Manual, SOP, Manual and Records
Project Requirements
Develop Project outline
Detailed list of applicable requirements including:
• Corporate and site Standard
• Good engineering practices
• Regulatory submission
• Application cGMP
• Heath, safety and Environmental
Approval of changes at any stage
Preform Project Review
Approved User Requirement specification
Approved Design specification
Approved Functional specification
Approved Installation specification
Approved Operation specification
Approved Performance specification
Approved Site Validation Master Plan
Category appropriate GAMP Development or Implementation life cycle
• User Requirement Specification
• Supplier Assessment
• Traceability Matrix
• Function Specification
• Design Specification
• Test Specification
• Quality plan
Organization Pillar
• Management Responsibilities Resources
• Manufacturing Operations
• Evaluation Activities
Validation
• Process Validation
• Cleaning Validation
• Software validation
• Hardware Validation
• Utility Validation
• Facility Validation
Life Cycle Approach
• New /Revised Site Layout Drawing
• Facility Layout Drawing
• Piping and instrument Drawing
• Equipment Layout
• Lux intensity Layout
• Man movement layout
• Equipment Movement Layout
• Safety Equipment Layout
• Current Calibration Certificates
• Certification for contract Substances
• Equipment, Calibration logs
• Spare Part list
• Maintenance Procedures
• Cleaning, Preventive maintenance Schedules
• Drain point layout
• Area and pressure classification layout
• Ducting layout
• Level of protection layout
• Fire detection and fire extinguisher system
• AHU grouping layout
• Grill layout
• Sampling point, water, steam air, Gases layout

CHAPTER 1

GMP Regulations for Pharmaceutical Industry

Introduction

A GMP is called as Good Manufacturing Practices and cGMP is called as current Good Manufacturing Practice. GMP is a system which ensuring that products are consistently produced and controlled according to quality standards and regulations, which protect the patient. GMP covers all aspects of production from the starting materials, premises and equipment to the training and personal hygiene of staff. Compliance with GMP is a necessary condition for the Marketing Authorization to sell the product. Standards are not legal rules they are guidelines, but nevertheless when linked to enforcement regimes and sanctions can be very powerful. cGMP always focus on Quality management, Quality assurance, Evaluation analysis, Quality risk management tools, Correction, Preventive action, Risk management and Continuous improvement.

1.1 Basic Requirements of GMP

(a) Manufacturing processes are clearly defined and controlled to ensure consistency and compliance with approved specifications.

(b) Critical steps of manufacturing processes and significant changes to the process are validated.

(c) Key elements for GMP including the following:

- Qualified and trained personnel,
- Adequate premises and space,
- Suitable equipment and services,
- Correct materials, containers and labels,

- Approved procedures and instructions,
- Suitable storage and transport.

(d) Instructions and procedures are written in clear and unambiguous language.

(e) Operators are trained to carry out and document procedures.

(f) Records are made during manufacture that demonstrate that all the steps required by the defined procedures and instructions were in fact taken and that the quantity and quality of the drug was as expected. Deviations are investigated and documented.

(g) Records of fabrication, packaging, labelling, testing, distribution, importation, and wholesaling that enable the complete history of a lot to be traced are retained in a comprehensible and accessible form.

(h) Control of storage, handling, and transportation of the drugs minimizes any risk to their quality.

(i) A system is available for recalling of drugs from sale.

(j) Complaints about drugs are examined, the causes of quality defects are investigated, and appropriate measures are taken with respect to the defective drugs and to prevent recurrence.

1. 2 Organization Pillars in cGMP

(a) ***Management responsibilities:*** Management play a key role in the design and implementation of quality system n cGMP. Leadership, structure organization, established policy, approved procedure, plan and review of system are root of the robust quality system.

(b) ***Resources:*** Senior management, or a designee is responsible for adequate resources such personnel, facilities, equipment, training, out sourcing activities, for robust quality system which involves in problem-solving and communicative organizational culture.

(c) ***Manufacturing operations:*** The product and process characteristics from design, development and commercial with input material, resource involved: facility, equipment and personnel, environment monitoring, monitoring of process and quality control testing.

(d) ***Evaluation activities:*** Continually monitoring trends and improving systems.

1.3 Six Quality System in GMP

Quality system is a centre hub which is connected to five other manufacturing subsystem such as Production System, Facilities and Equipment System, Laboratory Controls System, Materials System, Packaging and Labelling System. They are interlinked to each other to system is state of control.

A. Pharmaceutical Quality Management System

Quality management system a set of interaction elements designed to maintain the regulatory guideline, regulation, policies, resources, approved procedure, quality objective and risk assessment. It helps to develop an effective monitoring and continual improvement in product quality. Following are the aspects of:

- Defines the quality of product characteristics which have established identity, strength, purity, and potency.
- Product knowledge and process understanding from drug development to the commercial manufacturing.
- Quality Risk Management to mitigate the risk of changing a process or specification, and determine the extent of discrepancy investigations and corrective actions.
- CAPA (Corrective and Preventive Action): Remedial corrections of an identified problem, Root cause analysis with corrective action to help understand the cause of the deviation and potentially prevent recurrence of a similar problem and preventive action to avert recurrence of a similar potential problem.
- Focuses on managing change to prevent unintended consequences.
- Defines responsibility between quality control (QC) and quality assurance (QA) functions.

B. Production Management System

Production operations must be carried out accordance with the relevant manufacturing and marketing authorizations by competent people. All handling of materials and products, such as receipt and quarantine, sampling, storage, labelling, dispensing, processing, packaging and distribution must done as approved procedure. Real time documentation must be performed during each and every operation. Yield and reconciliation shall be carried out to check for acceptable limit. Operations on different products should not be carried out simultaneously or consecutively in the same room unless there is no risk of mix-up or cross-contamination. Risk assessment shall be carried out based on technical and organizational measures

a. **Technical Measures**

- Dedicated manufacturing facility (premises and equipment);
- Self-contained production areas having separate processing equipment and separate heating, ventilation and air-conditioning (HVAC) systems. It may also be desirable to isolate certain utilities from those used in other areas;
- Design of manufacturing process, premises and equipment to minimize opportunities for cross-contamination during processing, maintenance and cleaning;
- Use of "closed systems" for processing and material/product transfer between equipment;
- Use of physical barrier systems, including isolators, as containment measures;
- Controlled removal of dust close to source of the contaminant e.g. through localised extraction;
- Dedication of equipment, dedication of product contact parts or dedication of selected parts which are harder to clean (e.g. filters), dedication of maintenance tools;
- Use of single use disposable technologies;
- Use of equipment designed for ease of cleaning;
- Appropriate use of air-locks and pressure cascade to confine potential airborne contaminant within a specified area;
- Minimising the risk of contamination caused by recirculation or re-entry of untreated or insufficiently treated air;

- Use of automatic clean in place systems of validated effectiveness;
- For common general wash areas, separation of equipment washing, drying and storage areas.

b. Organisational Measures

- Dedicating the whole manufacturing facility or a self contained production area on a campaign basis (dedicated by separation in time) followed by a cleaning process of validated effectiveness;
- Keeping specific protective clothing inside areas where products with high risk of cross-contamination are processed;
- Cleaning verification after each product campaign should be considered as a detectability tool to support effectiveness of the Quality Risk Management approach for products deemed to present higher risk;
- Depending on the contamination risk, verification of cleaning of non product contact surfaces and monitoring of air within the manufacturing area and/or adjoining areas in order to demonstrate effectiveness of control measures against airborne contamination or contamination by mechanical transfer;
- Specific measures for waste handling, contaminated rinsing water and soiled gowning;
- Recording of spills, accidental events or deviations from procedures;
- Design of cleaning processes for premises and equipment such that the cleaning processes in themselves do not present a cross-contamination risk;
- Design of detailed records for cleaning processes to assure completion of cleaning in accordance with approved procedures and use of cleaning status labels on equipment and manufacturing areas;

- Use of common general wash areas on a campaign basis;
- Supervision of working behaviour to ensure training effectiveness and compliance with the relevant procedural controls.
- Measures to prevent cross-contamination and their effectiveness should be reviewed periodically according to set.

C. Facilities and Equipment Management System

Premises and equipment must be located, designed, constructed, adapted and maintained to suit the operations to be carried out. Their layout and design must aim to minimize the risk of errors and permit effective cleaning and maintenance in order to avoid cross-contamination, build-up of dust or dirt and, in general, any adverse effect on the quality of products. Facility and equipment must identify with specific number, qualify and validate at its operating range. Periodically check of facility and equipment must be carried out to check state of control. Equipment must adequately design and easily cleaned with its approved cleaning procedure. Calibration and Planned preventive maintenance program must be design. Pipelines and utilities must be mark with coding and direction. Defective equipment should, if possible, be removed from production and quality control areas, or at least be clearly labelled as defective.

D. Laboratory Controls Management System

Quality Control is concerned with sampling, specifications and testing as well as the organization,

Documentation and release procedures which ensure that the necessary and relevant tests are carried out and that materials are not released for use, nor products released for sale or supply, until their quality has been judged satisfactory. Quality Control is not confined to laboratory operations, but must be involved in all decisions which may concern the quality of the product. The independence of Quality Control from Production is considered fundamental to the satisfactory operation of Quality Control.

E. Materials Management System

Ware house areas must be designed to allow sufficient and orderly warehousing of various categories of materials and products like starting and packaging materials, intermediates, bulk and finished products, products in quarantine, released, rejected, returned or recalled, machine and equipment spare parts and change items. Ware house must be maintained clean free from rodent and environment control. It should separate loading and unloading bay protected from adverse whether, separated sampling and dispensing area.

- Highly hazardous, poisonous and explosive materials such as narcotics, psychotropic drugs and substances presenting potential risks of abuse, fire or explosion shall be stored in safe and secure areas.
- Printed packaging materials shall be stored in safe, separate and secure area.
- Separate dispensing areas for β (Beta) lactum, Sex hormones and Cytotoxic substances or any such special categories of product shall be provided with proper supply of filtered air and suitable measures for dust control to avoid contamination. Such areas shall be under differential pressure.
- Sampling and dispensing of sterile materials shall be conducted under aseptic conditions conforming to Grade A, which can also be performed in a dedicated area within the manufacturing facility.
- Regular checks shall be made to ensure adequate steps are taken against spillage, breakage and leakage of containers.
- FIFO (Frist in first out) and FEFO (Frist expiry first out) inventory management.
- Inventory management

F. Packaging and Labelling Management System

Packaging and labeling concerned about label affixed to the product which gives identity to the product. The label manufacturer is responsible for making sure that the print is legible and will remain that way throughout the product's life span. Every label printed should be inspected thoroughly to ensure the information is consistent and accurate. The products should be separated to prevent any mix-ups or switches. Product separation can be physical or spatial, or can be completed by performing press runs at different times to avoid confusion. Proper storage control is necessary for preventing any mix-ups or switches when dealing with labels printed for use in the pharmaceutical industry

Before packaging operations are begun,

- Ensure that the work area, packaging lines, printing machines and other equipment are clean and free from any products, materials or documents previously used.
- Correct product name batch number on each packing station line.
- The line-clearance must be performed according to an appropriate check-list. All products and packaging materials quantity to be used should be checked for code number, retest date and expiry date.
- Re-checked at regular intervals.
- Special care should be taken when using cut-labels and when over-printing is carried out off-line. Roll-feed labels are normally preferable to cut-labels, in helping to avoid mix-ups.
- Electronic code readers, label counters or similar devices are operating correctly.
- Printed and embossed information on packaging materials should be distinct and resistant to fading or erasing.
- On-line control of the product during packaging should include at least checking the following:

    a. General appearance of the packages;
    b. Whether the packages are complete;
    c. Whether the correct products and packaging materials are used;
    d. Whether any over-printing is correct;
    e. Correct functioning of line monitors.

- Samples taken away from the packaging line should not be returned.

  Upon completion of a packaging operation, any unused batch-coded packaging materials should be destroyed and the destruction recorded. A documented procedure should be followed if un-coded printed materials are returned to stock.

1. 4 Quality Culture and Pharmaceutical Industry

Culture means core value, guide, principles, behaviors and Attitudes. Quality culture in an organization is drives through the policies, practices, and processes used to accomplish an organization's work. Quality culture can build by understanding organization environment.

Who we are? Where we are? Where we want to reach? How we can do?

The culture of an organization is the embodiment of the core values, guiding principles, behaviors, and attitudes that collectively contribute to its daily operations. Culture drives the policies, practices, and processes used to accomplish an organization's work.

Quality culture will be developed by transparent and open by communicating the information at all level. An organization shall create a work environment transparent and open, one in which personnel are encouraged to freely communicate failures and mistakes, including potential data reliability issues, so that corrective and preventative actions can be taken.

An organization can foster quality culture by:

- Trust among each and every employee
- Code of Ethics and Code of Conduct: Not on paper base. By understanding and awareness for personnel.
- An organization should demonstrate the behaviors they expect to see from top to low management.
- Ensure accountability for actions and decisions.
- Stay continuously and actively involved.
- Set realistic expectations, consider the limitations that place pressures on employees.
- Allocate resources to meet expectations.

- Implement fair and just consequences and rewards and
- Be aware of regulatory trends to apply lessons learned to your organization.
- Investigation programs and problem solving and Review practice.
- Training program and decision making and Regular management review of quality metrics.
- Resource allocation, Team spirit, Role models.
- Continuous improvements and motivation.
- It is the collection of values, beliefs, thinking, and behaviors demonstrated consistently by management, team leaders, quality personnel and all personnel that contribute to creating a quality culture in an organization.

CHAPTER 2

Good Laboratory Practices in Pharmaceutical Industry

Introduction

GLP refers to a quality system to ensure the uniformity, consistency, reliability, reproducibility, quality and integrity of the data. GLP gives true reflection of tested results. Good laboratory practice must be planned, reliable, accurate, recorded, reported, monitor and archive all data generated during analysis or testing. The purpose of testing items is to obtain information on their safety with respect to human health and environment. GLP is also required for registration purpose and licensing of pharmaceuticals, pesticides, food additives, veterinary drug products and some bio-products.

Personnel working in laboratory must have education, training, and experience, or combination thereof, to enable that individual to perform the assigned functions. Facilities must be adequate and environment control.

2.1 Good Laboratory Practice Equipment

- *Design:* Equipment's used for generation, measurements and assessments of study data shall be of appropriate design and capacity. They shall be suitably located for operation, inspection and maintenance. Validation and Qualification of equipment's must be done to make sure that consistent intended functions are performed.
- *Maintenance:* Cleaning and maintenance of equipment's is very critical. They must be adequately tested, calibrated and standardized. The entire process is called qualification for equipment's. Time interval for calibration, re-validation and testing of equipment's depends on the equipment itself, laboratory experience and extent of use.

- *Records and other documents:* Written records shall be maintained for qualification of equipment's and validation operations including date of operation, and specify is SOP s were followed for conducting maintenance operation. These equipment records can be maintained in the form of a log book

2.2 Documentation in Good Laboratory Practice

- Specifications.
- Procedures describing sampling, testing, records (including test worksheets and/or laboratory notebooks), recording and verifying.
- Procedures for and records of the calibration/qualification of instruments and maintenance of equipment.
- A procedure for the investigation of Out of Specification and Out of Trend results.
- Testing reports and/or certificates of analysis.
- Data from environmental (air, water and other utilities) monitoring, where required.
- Validation records of test methods, where applicable.
- Trend analysis for test results and environment controls.
- All raw data such as laboratory notebooks and/or records should be retained and readily available.

2.3 Sampling in Good Laboratory Practice

- Sampling may be required for different purposes, such as prequalification; acceptance of consignments; batch release testing in-process control; special controls; inspection for customs clearance, deterioration or adulteration; or for obtaining a retention sample. Sampling shall consist following contents:
- Approved procedure, Sampling plans and methods must be written and defined.
- Samples must be representative of the population.
- Samples or sampling plans must be based on appropriate statistical criteria, and
- Representative of batch.
- Sample should be Samples must be properly identified and handled.

- Equipment to be used the amount of the sample to be taken;
- Instructions for any required sub-division of the sample;
- The type and condition of the sample container to be used;
- Identification of containers sampled,
- Any special precautions to be observed, especially with regard to the sampling of sterile or noxious materials; storage conditions;
- Instructions for the cleaning and storage of sampling equipment.

A. Approaches for sampling plans will be discussed for:

- Incoming Packaging Components
- Incoming Raw Materials
- Labeling Materials
- Non-sterile Liquid Products
- Sterile Products
- Creams, Suspensions, and Emulsions
- Powder Blends
- Tablets, Capsules, and Other Solid Dosage Forms

2.4 Testing in Good Laboratory Practice

Testing methods should be validated. A laboratory that is using a testing method and which are defined in the marketing authorization or technical dossier. The results obtained should be recorded. The tests performed should be recorded and the records should include at least the following data:

- Name of the material or product and, where applicable, dosage form;
- Batch number and, where appropriate, the manufacturer and/or supplier;
- References to the relevant specifications and testing procedures;
- Test results, including observations and calculations, and reference to any certificates of analysis;
- Dates of testing;
- Initials of the persons who performed the testing;
- Initials of the persons who verified the testing and the calculations, where appropriate;

- A clear statement of approval or rejection (or other status decision) and the dated signature of the designated responsible person;
- Reference to the equipment used.

2.5 Laboratory Reagents, Solutions, Reference Standards and Culture Media in Good Laboratory Practice

- Laboratory reagents, solutions, reference standards and culture media should be marked with the preparation and opening date and the signature of the person who prepared them. The expiry date of reagents and culture media should be indicated on the label, together with specific storage conditions. In addition, for volumetric solutions, the last date of standardization and the last current factor should be indicated.
- Qualified Reference standards must be suitable for their intended use. Qualification and certification should be clearly stated and documented. Whenever compendial reference standards from an officially recognized source exist, these should preferably be used as primary reference standards unless fully justified (the use of secondary standards is permitted once their traceability to primary standards has been demonstrated and is documented). These compendial materials should be used for the purpose described in the appropriate monograph unless otherwise authorized by the National Competent Authority.
- Culture media should be prepared in accordance with the media manufacturer's requirements unless scientifically justified. The performance of all culture media should be verified prior to use.
- Used microbiological media and strains should be decontaminated according to a standard procedure and disposed of in a manner to prevent the cross-contamination and retention of residues. The in-use shelf life of microbiological media should be established, documented and scientifically justified.
- Animals used for testing components, materials or products, should, where appropriate, be quarantined before use. They should be maintained and controlled in a manner that assures their suitability for the intended use. They should be identified, and adequate records should be maintained, showing the history of their use.

2.6 Glassware in Good Laboratory Practice

Glass used for pharmaceutical containers is either borosilicate (neutral) glass or soda-lime-silica glass. Class A apparatus are directly used for analysis based on the calibration certificate. Class B apparatus must be calibrated by in house approved method.

2.7 On-going Stability Programme in Good Laboratory Practice

The on-going stability programme is to monitor the product over its shelf life and to determine that the product remains, and can be expected to remain, within specifications under the labelled storage conditions. The on-going stability programme should be described in a written protocol and should include, but not be limited to, the following parameters:

- Number of batch(es) per strength and different batch sizes, if applicable;
- Relevant physical, chemical, microbiological and biological test methods;
- Acceptance criteria;
- Reference to test methods;
- Description of the container closure system(s);
- Testing intervals (time points);
- Description of the conditions of storage (standardised ICH/VICH conditions for long term testing, consistent with the product labelling, should be used);
- Other applicable parameters specific to the medicinal product.

The number of batches and frequency of testing should provide a sufficient amount of data to allow for trend analysis. Unless otherwise justified, at least one batch per year of product manufactured in every strength and every primary packaging type, if relevant, should be included in the stability programme (unless none are produced during that year). For products where on-going stability monitoring would normally require testing using animals and no appropriate alternative, validated techniques are available, the frequency of testing may take account of a risk-benefit approach. The principle of bracketing and matrixing designs may be applied if scientifically justified in the protocol. In certain situations, additional batches should be included in the on-going stability programme. For example, an on-going stability study should be conducted after any significant change or significant deviation to the process or package. Any reworking, reprocessing or recovery operation should also be considered for inclusion.

2.8 Technical Transfer of Testing Methods in Good Laboratory Practice

Priorto transferring a test method, the transferring site should verify that the test method(s) comply with those as described in the Marketing Authorization or the relevant technical dossier. The transfer of testing methods from one laboratory (transferring laboratory) to another laboratory (receiving laboratory) should be described in a detailed protocol. The transfer protocol should include, but not be limited to, the following parameters:

- Identification of the testing to be performed and the relevant test method(s) under going transfer.
- Identification of the additional training requirements.
- Identification of standards and samples to be tested.
- Identification of any special transport and storage conditions of test items.
- The acceptance criteria which should be based upon the current validation study.
- Deviations from the protocol should be investigated prior to closure of the technical transfer process.
- The technical transfer report should document the comparative outcome of the process and should identify areas requiring further test method revalidation, if applicable.

2.9 Measures in Good Laboratory Practice

- ***Establish and follow procedures:*** Develop approved procedures and inventory.
- ***Maintain your proficiency:*** Analysts must have the education, training and experience, acquired through formal education or on-the-job training, sufficient to perform assigned analytic duties.
- ***Validate methods:*** Method should be validated before usages.
- ***Use traceable standard reference materials (SRM):*** Reference material uses include validating methods that help ensure

accurate data from individual test runs, calibrating instruments and assessing analyst proficiency. In the United States, a NIST standard reference material is considered the "gold standard" for that material. NIST has more than a thousand different SRMs covering diverse technologies. The results of analyses backed by NIST-traceable SRMs are widely accepted as valid.

- ***Run in duplicate:*** The purpose of duplicate (sometimes triplicate) testing is to add to the confidence that the test run has produced good data for the test object. Replicate data that is in agreement is a good measure of method reproducibility but does not prove data accuracy (validity).
- ***Keep original data:*** Document everything and Maintain Good Records. Whether data is first recorded in electronic/digital form, in a notebook or on the closest piece of scrap paper, keep it.
- ***Assign instruments and equipment to analysts:*** A good practice is to formally assign that analyst the responsibility for keeping the instrument operational and for alerting management to malfunctions. When an instrument is used by multiple staff members, assign these responsibilities to a primary user, who should schedule usage time for other staff members, provide training and mentoring to new users, ensure that any instrument control charts are current and ensure that calibration and maintenance occur on schedule.
- ***Calibrate instruments and equipment:*** Instrument should be calibrated to its working range.
- ***Use control charts:*** **Control** charts are excellent tools for several uses, including those already noted. A control chart enables a laboratory to track the results of a reference material and/or control sample at the end of each test run. It gives the laboratory a snapshot of test run quality and a picture of the quality of the laboratory's results for that particular test over time.

CHAPTER 3

Good Microbiology Practice in Pharmaceutical Industry

Introduction

Good laboratory practices in a microbiology laboratory consist of activities that depend on several principles: aseptic technique, control of media, control of test strains, operation and control of equipment, diligent recording and evaluation of data, and training of the laboratory staff. Because of the inherent risk of variability in microbiology data, reliability and reproducibility are dependent on the use of accepted methods and adherence to good laboratory practices.

3.1 Premises, Layout and Zone

Microbiology laboratory generally divided into clean or aseptic areas and live culture areas. If complete separation of live and clean culture zones cannot be accomplished, then other barriers (such as protective clothing, sanitization and disinfection procedures, and biological safety cabinets designated for clean or aseptic operations only) and aseptic practices should be employed to reduce the likelihood of accidental contamination. Areas in which environmental or sterile product samples are handled and incubated should be maintained completely free of live cultures, if possible. Separate air supply, air handling unit should be available for laboratories and production areas. Sterility testing should always be performed in a dedicated area. Access to the microbiological laboratory should be restricted to authorized personnel.

Laboratory activities, such as sample preparation, media and equipment preparation and enumeration of microorganisms, should be segregated by space or at least time, so as to minimize risks of cross-contamination and false positives. Where non-dedicated arras are used, risk management principles should be applied.

Operations should be carried out preferably in the following zones:

Zone	Installation Grade	Proposed
Sample receipt	Unclassified	Unclassified
Media preparation	Unclassified	Unclassified
Autoclave loading inside the sterility testing area	Grade B	ISO 5 (turbulent) and <10 cfu/m^3
Sterility testing – UDAF	Grade A	ISO 5 (UDAF) &<1 cfu/m^3
Sterility testing – backdround to UDAF	Grade B	ISO 5 (UDAF) &<10 cfu/m^3
Sterility testing-Isolator	Grade A(NVP and microbiology only)	ISO 5(UDAF) and < 1cfu/m^3
Sterility Testing-Background to isolator	Unclassified	Unclassified
Incubator	Unclassified	Unclassified
Enumerration	*Unclassified	*Unclassified
Decontamination	Unclassified	Unclassified
cfu, colony-forming unit. *A Critical steps should be done under laminar flow.		

3.2 Laboratory Environmental Monitoring

Appropriate an environmental monitoring programme should be in place i.e use of air settlement plates and surface swabbing, temperature and pressure differentials. Alert and action limits should be defined. Trending of environmental monitoring results shall be carried out.

3.3 Laboratory Equipment

Each item of equipment, instrument or other device used for testing, verification and calibration should be uniquely identified and should have a documented programme for the maintenance, calibration and monitoring of its equipment.

Laboratory equipment used in the microbiology laboratory should not be used outside the microbiology area, unless there are specific precautions in place to prevent cross-contamination.

3.4 Personnel

Each person engaged in laboratory should have the education, training, and experience to do his or her job. Thet should have basic training in microbiology and relevant practical experience before being allowed to perform work covered by the scope of testing. Personnel should be made aware of:

(a) the appropriate entry and exit procedures including gowning;

(b) the intended use of a particular area;

(c) the restrictions imposed on working within such areas;

(d) the reasons for imposing such restrictions; and

(e) the appropriate containment levels.

3.5 Media and Preparation

A. *Media procurement and storage:* Media should be purchase from be approved and qualified vendor. Media should be clearly labeled with batch or lot numbers, preparation and expiration dates, and media identification. Each media should consist of a certificate of analysis describing expiration dating and recommended storage conditions, as well as the quality control organisms used in growth-promotion and selectivity testing of that media. Growth promotion should be done on all media on every batch by the user. Media should always be storage under validated controlled condition to ensure its quality through to the expiry date and also to minimize the loss of moisture, control the temperature, prevent microbial contamination, and provide mechanical protection to the prepared media.

B. *Media preparation:* Media should be prepared as per manufacture formula, instruction for routine dehydrated media and ready-made media preparation. Cleaned container and tools should be used for preparation of the media to prevent foreign substance entering in the preparation. Equipment used in the preparation of media should be appropriate to allow for controlled heating, constant agitation, and mixing of the media. Darkening of media is generally indication of overheating of media. Sterilization of media should be performed within the parameters provided by the manufacturer or validated by the user. Remelting of an original container of solid media should be performed only once to avoid media whose quality is compromised by overheating or potential contamination. It is recommended that remelting be performed in a heated water bath or by using free-flowing steam. The pH of each batch of medium should be confirmed by a flat pH probe at room temperature (20°–25°) by aseptically withdrawing a sample for testing. The pH of media should be in a range of ± 0.2 of the value indicated by the manufacturer, unless a wider range is acceptable by the validated method.

Prepared media should be checked by appropriate inspection of plates and tubes for the following:

(a) Cracked containers or lids
(b) Unequal filling of containers
(c) Dehydration resulting in cracks or dimpled surfaces on solid medium
(d) Hemolysis
(e) Excessive darkening or color change
(f) Crystal formation from possible freezing
(g) Excessive number of bubbles
(h) Microbial contamination
(i) Status of redox indicators (if appropriate)
(j) Lot number and expiration date checked and recorded
(k) Sterility of the media
(l) Cleanliness of plates (lid should not stick to dish)

Growth promotion test should be performed on each lot prepared media based on manufacturer recommendation micro-organism or may include representative environmental isolates (but these latter are not to be construed as compendial requirements). Expiration dates on media should have supporting growth-promotion testing to indicate that the performance of the media still meets acceptance criteria up to and including the expiration date. The length of shelf life of a batch of media will depend on the stability of the ingredients and formulation under specified conditions, as well as the type of container and closure. Disposal of used cultured media (as well as expired media) should follow local biological hazard safety procedures.

C. ***Media incubation time:*** Incubation times for microbiological tests of less than 3 days' duration should be expressed in hours: e.g.,

"Incubate at 30°to 35° for 18 to 72 hours". Tests longer than 72 hours' duration should be expressed in days: e.g., "Incubate at 30° to 35° for 3 to 5 days". For incubation times expressed in hours, incubate for the minimum specified time, and exercise good microbiological judgment when exceeding the incubation time.

3.6 Reference Culture

Cultures for use in compendial tests should be acquired from a national culture collection or a qualified secondary supplier. They can be acquired frozen, freeze-dried, on slants, or in ready-to-use forms. Confirmation of the purity of the culture and the identity of the culture should be performed before its use in quality control testing. Ready-to-use cultures should be subjected to incoming testing for purity and identity before use. The confirmation of identity for commonly used laboratory strains should ideally be done at the level of genus and species. All cultures must be no more than 5 passages removed from the original stock culture. The number of transfers of working control cultures should be tracked to prevent excessive sub culturing that increases the risk of phenotypic alteration or mutation. Working stocks shall not be subculture to replace reference stocks. Reference strains may only be used as working cultures. Test culture are :

(a) Candida albicans (ATCC No. 10231)
(b) Aspergillus brasiliensis (ATCC No. 16404) (formerly Aspergillus niger)
(c) Escherichia coli (ATCC No. 8739)
(d) Pseudomonas aeruginosa (ATCC No. 9027)
(e) Staphylococcus aureus (ATCC No. 6538)

3.7 Sampling

Sampling should only be performed by trained personnel. It should be carried out aseptically using sterile equipment. Appropriate precautions should be taken to ensure that sample integrity is maintained through the use of sterile sealed containers for the collection of samples where appropriate. It may be necessary to monitor environmental conditions for instance air contamination and temperature at the sampling site. Time of sampling should be recorded. The laboratory should record all relevant information, e.g.:

(a) date and, where relevant, the time of receipt;

(b) condition of the sample on receipt and, when necessary, temperature; and

(c) characteristics of the sampling operation (sampling date, sampling conditions, etc.).

3.8 Laboratory Testing

All testing in laboratories used for critical testing procedures, such as sterility testing of final dosage forms, bulk product, seed cultures for biological production, or cell cultures used in biological production, should be performed under controlled conditions. Isolator technology is also appropriate for critical, sterile microbiological testing. Isolators have been shown to have lower levels of environmental contamination than manned clean rooms, and therefore, are generally less likely to produce false-positive results. Proper validation of isolators is critical both to ensure environmental integrity and to prevent the possibility of false-negative results as a result of chemical disinfection of materials brought into or used within isolators Subculturing, staining, microbial identification, or other investigational operations should be undertaken in the live culture section of the laboratory. If possible, any sample found to contain growing colonies should not be opened in the clean zone of the laboratory. Careful segregation of contaminated samples and materials will reduce false-positive results.

Staff engaged in sampling activities should not enter or work in the live culture handling section of a laboratory unless special precautions are taken, including wearing protective clothing and gloves and careful sanitizing of hands upon exiting.

All test performed should be document as and when performed.

Discrepancy and failure investigations related to manufacturing and testing: documented; evaluated; investigated in a timely manner; includes corrective action where appropriate.

3.9 Disposal of Contaminated Waste

The procedures for the disposal of contaminated materials should be designed to minimize the possibility of contaminating the test environment or materials. It is a matter of good laboratory management and should conform to national/international environmental or health and safety regulations.

3.10 Laboratory Data Management

All laboratory records should be archived and protected against catastrophic loss. A formal record retention and retrieval program should be in place.

- Microbiologist training and verification of proficiency.
- Equipment validation, calibration, and maintenance.
- Equipment performance during test (e.g., 24-hour/7-day chart recorders).
- Media preparation, sterility checks, and growth-promotion and selectivity capabilities.
- Media inventory and control testing.
- Critical aspects of test conducted as specified by a procedure.
- Data and calculations verification.
- Reports reviewed by qualified responsible manager.
- Investigation of data deviations (when required).
- Test results should include the original plate counts, allowing a reviewer to recreate the calculations used to derive the final test results.
- If charts or graphs are incorporated into laboratory notebooks, they should be secured with clear tape and should not be obstructing any data on the page. The chart or graph should be signed by the person adding the document, with the signature overlapping the chart and the notebook page.
- Lab notebooks should include page numbers, a table of contents for reference, and an intact timeline of use.
- The laboratory write-up should include Date, Material tested, Microbiologist's name, Procedure number, Document test results, Deviations (if any), Documented parameters (equipment used, microbial stock cultures used, media lots used) and Management/Second review signature.

CHAPTER 4

Good Aseptic Practices in Pharmaceutical Industry

Introduction

Expedient risk assessment of aseptic manufacturing processes offers unique opportunities for improved and sustained assurance of product quality. This article reviews current industry practices and regulatory expectations for the aseptic processing of sterile drugs. It provides comparisons and outlines points of tension between current manufacturing. Technology and capabilities with regulatory "requirements" for this important activity.

4.1 The Industry's Approach to Validation of Aseptic Manufacturing

Comprehensive engineering qualifications are conducted on each new sterilizer to ensure that the design and functional specifications are met. These qualification activities are used as the basis for formalized change control programs that support the continued appropriateness of the sterilizer over time. In addition, the maintenance procedures and calibration requirements for all process control devices are developed, as are the necessary standard operating procedures for these activities. Following completion of the qualification of the sterilizer, process validation is undertaken to ensure that the sterilization process complies with regulatory requirements. A risk based approach should be considered throughout the qualification phases.

Validation typically includes an adequate margin of safety to allow for process variation. After the prospective validation has been completed, change control systems are established to ensure that sterilizers are maintained in a state of control. In addition to periodic performance checks, calibration, and maintenance checks, is done to ensure that no change is made to any aspect of the sterilization process.

Process validation must be completed prior to the distribution and sale of the medicinal product. Revalidation of the process should be addresses regarding each specific situations to guarantee that the process remain valid, considering the situation when process modification occurs.

4.2 Cleanroom Classification

The classification of each room or module within an aseptic processing area must be appropriate for its intended use. The highest level of control will be directed to those areas, typically known as critical zones, in which aseptic manipulation of uncovered containers, closures, or components occurs. These areas are designed to comply with Class 5 of ISO 14644 (ISO Class 5 is functionally equivalent to traditional US Federal Standard (FS) 209 E Class 100, and to EU Grade A)(12, 21, 22).

Parameters that must be evaluated when testing a cleanroom: Leak test to the HEPA filter, number of particles, air changes rate, recovery time of the cleanroom after a contamination event, air flow pattern and pressure differentials.

4.3 Environmental Monitoring

According to EU Guide11 sampling is required at the end of a critical processing step to avoid any risk from the product. FDA Guidance24 requires measurements during the whole process. The USP determines intervals of sampling (each operating shift for Class A or better and B; twice / a week for class C in case of product contact; once / a week in case of non-product-contact). But nothing is said regarding the number of sampling points.

4.4 Methods of Microbiological Monitoring

There are different methods and equipment available for testing air, surfaces and personnel.

4.5 Microbial Identification

Microorganisms that are isolated during routine environmental monitoring are characterized by their cellular morphology and staining reactions as gram-positive rods, cocci, and rod-shaped spore-formers; gram-negative bacteria; or identified by genus or species depending on the criticality of the sampling location with respect to product exposure. Genotypic microbial identification methods may be less subjective, less dependent on the culture method, and theoretically more reliable than phenotypic methods because nucleic acid are highly conserved by species.

4.6 Identification of Isolates

Clean Room Class	Exceeding Limit Investigation
Class A /Class B/ Class C	**Action** limit: Identification of all morphologically different colonies
	Alert limit / no exceeding limit: Shortened identification of all morphologically different colonies. Class C: Addition to above; if there is a suspicion of Pseudomonas or spore generating germs

4.7 Essential Elements of the Environmental Control and Facility Management Program

The basic elements of an aseptic processing environmental control program have not changed

- A review of environmental factors that generally include temperature, relative humidity, air velocity, unidirectional air flow, HEPA filtration, and pressure differentials between rooms of different classification.
- An evaluation of utility services that could affect microbiological safety or product quality.
- A comprehensive microbiological and total-particulate monitoring system.
- An evaluation of personnel gowning and materials transfer airlocks.
- Calibration, certification and preventive maintenance on critical facility, systems and processing equipment.
- Training programs for personnel in both aseptic technique and operating procedures/work instructions.
- These systems should subject to regular scheduled/unscheduled audits, routine supervisory oversight and evaluation.

4.8 Training for Aseptic Operations

The proper training of personnel involved in aseptic processing is crucial. Training provides assurance that jobs are done correctly. A training can be conducted by a single or combination of different methods. Gowning Training and Behavior Training plays important role in aseptic area. Gowning training must be thorough and offer the operator plenty of time to practice and become proficient and ensure the technician is ready for gowning qualification tests.

Behavior training shall consist Aerodynamic position, where the palms are facing HEPA air so they are constantly bathed with clean, non-contaminated air flow, Walking versus remaining stationary, Walking movements, Always minimalize movements and talking, Any movements must be slow and deliberate .

4.9 Process Simulating Testing

The most challenging issue, when validating a sterile process is the microbiological contamination control and expected to guarantee zero contamination. To demonstrate, stimulation process is done using nutrient media instead of real product, is usually called as media fill. When designing the stimulation test, it is necessary to select worst case scenarios. Risk assessment tools are useful to help determine the validation process.

Approved protocol should include the information such as process simulation test, identification of process, operator number, and numbers of container to be filled. Type of container, speed of the filling line, type and amount of media fill, duration of filling, environmental monitoring, acceptance criteria, incubation condition, rejection units and results.

1. **Production batch size (Containers) <5000 and Size of production batch <5000**
    - No contamination unit should be detected.
    - One (1) contaminated unit-investigation & revalidation
2. **Production batch size (Containers) ≥ 5000:**
    (a) Minimum Containers tested per Run: 5000-10000
    - One (1) contaminated unit-investigation & repeated media fill.
    - Two (2) contaminated unit-investigation & revalidation.

(b) Minimum Containers tested per Run: ≥10000

- One (1) contaminated unit-investigation.
- Two (2) contaminated unit-investigation & revalidation.

4.10 Measure of Good Aseptic Practices

Sterile drug product manufacturing continues to be a concern by regulators and industry. Recently warning letter were issued due to practices in Media fill, Personnel, Microbiology laboratory, Clean room qualification, Environment monitoring, Disinfectant qualification, Visual inspection Investigation and sterilization of equipment. Effective and innovative control strategies must be designed and in place to reduce the risk of process failure. The most effective way to assure sterile drug product quality is through sound process design which identifies process variables, evaluates their relative risk, and reduces or controls their effect on product quality. Training also play important role in manufacturing of drugs.

CHAPTER 5

Good Clean Room Monitoring in Pharmaceutical Industry

Introduction

Both the European and US FDA cGMP documents refer ISO 14644-1 as the method for cleanroom classification/qualification. ISO 14644-1 was revised and re-issued in December 2015, impacting immediately on GMP cleanroom users. The challenge for pharmaceutical companies is that they will now have to revise their cleanroom validation/requalification programs to meet the requirements of the new ISO 14644-1:2015. An additional challenge is that ISO 14644-1:2015 requires that the air particle counters used for cleanroom classification/qualification must meet the performance standard ISO 21501-4:2007 and many older particle counters simply will not pass the exacting requirements of this performance standard. Pharmaceutical companies will need to plan to replace older particle counters with ISO21501-4:2007 compliant models. The newly updated ISO14644-1:2015 has caused some confusion want to be ensure to address expectation. This GMP arsenal focus and requirements and implementation of ISO 14644-1:2015. Before implementation of new guidelines one should assess the question such as what is sampling Locations, Risk Analysis, Cleanroom Monitoring, Class and Limits, ISO 21501 and Calibration, ISO Technical Committee TC-209, Particle Counters and Applications.

Two Key Changes to ISO 14644-1:

- The first major change in ISO14644-1:2015 is the requirement to follow ISO 21501-4, which defines **calibration and performance requirements of air particle counters**. Many older air particle counters currently in use do not comply with this new requirement.

- **Secondly, the number of required sample locations for the cleanroom validation/qualification process has increased significantly.** The larger number of required samples vastly increases the number of associated paper records and manual data transcriptions and the subsequent risk of data loss/transcription errors.
- As a result of these changes, all GMP cleanroom users will have to make changes to their cleanroom classification/re-qualification procedures to meet the requirements laid out in the new version of ISO 14644-1. Furthermore, it is possible that the required new classification sampling plan may affect the reported cleanroom class and some cleanroom owners may have to make changes to their cleanroom and the HVAC system to return to the required Class/Grade.
    - (a) The classification number, expressed as "ISO Class N (Nine ISO cleanliness classes at rest.
    - (b) **ISO 14644-1Principle:** Specifies classes of air cleanliness in term of the number of particles expressed as a concentration in air volume.

Area of cleanroom (m2) less than or equal to	Min number of SL to be tested (NL)
2	1
4	2
6	3
8	4
10	5
24	6
28	7
32	8
36	9
52	10
56	11
64	12
68	13
72	14
76	15
104	16
108	17
116	18
148	19
156	20
192	21
232	22

Table *Contd...*

<table>
<tr><th>Area of cleanroom (m2) less than or equal to</th><th>Min number of SL to be tested (NL)</th></tr>
<tr><td>276</td><td>23</td></tr>
<tr><td>352</td><td>24</td></tr>
<tr><td>436</td><td>25</td></tr>
<tr><td>636</td><td>26</td></tr>
<tr><td>1000</td><td>27</td></tr>
<tr><td>>1000</td><td>See Formula (A.1)</td></tr>
<tr><td colspan="2">• Area falls between two values in table, the greater of the two should be selected.
• In case of unidirectional airflow, the area may be considered as the cross section of the moving air perpendicular to the direction of the airflow. In all other case the area may be considered as the horizontal plan area of the clean room.
• Area greater than 1000m^2,apply formula (A.1) to determine the minimum number of sampling locations N_l+27 X (A/1000)</td></tr>
</table>

5.1 Content of ISO 14644-1:2015

- **Parts 1: Classification** of air cleanliness by particle.
- **Parts 2: Monitoring** to provide evidence of cleanroom related to air cleanliness by particle concentration.
- **Parts 3: Test** methods.
- **Parts 4: Design**, construction and stat-up.
- **Parts 5: Operations.**
- **Parts 7: Separate device** (clean air hoods, glove boxes, isolators and mini-environments.
- **Parts 8: Classification** of air cleanliness by chemical concentration.
- **Parts 9: Classification** of surface cleanliness by particle concentration.
- **Parts 10: Classification** of surface cleanliness by chemical concentration (ACC).

5.2 Sampling and Location Evaluations

Statistical Approach for selection and evaluation the number of sampling location is adopted which is based on hypergeometric sampling model techniques. Samples are drawn randomly without replacement from a finite population. Each location is treated independently with at least a 95% level of confidence that at least 90% of the cleanroom area will comply with the maximum particle concentration limit for target class. No assumption are made regarding the distribution of the actual particle counts over the area of cleanroom. Sampling location shall be selected from Table A which defines the minimum number of sampling locations .The clean room is divided into grids of sections of near equal area, whose number is equal to the number of sampling location derived from Table A.

5.3 Sampling

Sampling location is placed within each grid section, so as to be representative of each grid. Representative sample location means the feature such as clean room/zone layout, equipment disposition and airflow systems should be considered when selecting sampling location. Addition sampling point may be included to minimum number of sampling location considering criticality and sub divide in equal section. For non-unidirectional airflow cleanrooms/ zones, location may not be representative if they are located directly beneath non-diffused supply air source.

5.4 Sampling Procedure

Set particle counter at zero count set. Sample shall collected directly from the air at the sampling location. On-unidirectional airflow exits, the probe should be located with the sample inlet facing vertically upward. Use inlet of sampling probe directed vertical upward where air flow is not controlled or non-unidirectional. Sample volume of air sufficient to detect minimum 20 particles (at least 2L with a minimum sampling time of 1 min.

5.5 Sampling Instruments: LSAPC – Light Scattering Airborne Particle Counter

Test instrument (LSAPC) shall meets specification given in ISO 21501-4: 2007.

- Valid calibration certification.
- Sample flow rate of a least 28.03 L/min.
- Should fitted with an inlet probe sized for isokinetic sampling in unidirectional flow zone.
- Transit tube length should be exceed longer than 1 m in length. Minimum sampling error.

- LSAPC particle size range setting shall be done one size below 5 μm, to ensure that the concentration of detected particles below the macro particle size is not sufficiently high to cause coincidence error. The particle concentration in lower size range, when added to the macro particles concentration, should not exceed 50% of the maximum recommended particle concentration specified for the LSAPC being used.

5.6 Recording and Evaluations of Airborne Particle Concentration

Single sample volume at each location shall not exceed the concentration limit. If multiple single sample volume are taken at a sampling location, the concentrations shall be average and average concentration must not exceed the concentration limits.

5.7 ISO Class Number

ISO class number (N)	Maximum allowable concentrations(particles/m³) for particles equal to and greater than the considered sizes, shown below[a]					
	0.1 μm	0.2μm	0.3μm	0.5 μm	1μm	5μm
1	10 [b]	D	D	D	d	e
2	100	24 [b]	10 [b]	D	d	e
3	1000	237	102	35[b]	D	e
4	10000	2370	1020	352	83 [b]	e
5	100000	23700	10200	3520	832	d,e,f
6	1000000	237000	102000	35200	8320	293
7	C	C	C	352000	83200	2930
8	C	C	C	3520000	832000	29300
9g	C	C	C	35200000	8320000	29300

a. All concentrations in the table are cumulative, e.g. For ISO Class 5, 10200 particles at 0.3 um include all Particles equal to and greater than this size.

b. These concentrations will lead to larger air sample volumes for classification.

c. Concentration limits are not applicable in this region of the table due to very high particle concentration

d. Sampling and statistical limitations for particles in low concentrations make classification in appropriate.

e. Sample collection limitations for both particles in low concentrations and sizes greater than 1 u make classification at this particle size in appropriate, due to potential particle losses in the sampling system.

f. In order to specify this particle size in association with ISO class 5, the macro particle descriptor M may be adapted and in conjunction with at least one other particles size.

g. This class is only applicable for the in-operation.

GMP (EU/PICs/WHO) Should use the macro-particle concept for

Grade A :	Grade B (rest) :	ISO M
20 particles/m³ ≥ 5.0 μ	29 particles /m ³ ≥ 5.0 μ	(20; ≥ 5.0 μ) LSAPC
M = Macro Particles	20 = Class GMP lit	5.0 = Consider particle size

LSAPAC=Light scattering airborne particle counter

5.8 Test Reports and Interpretation of Results

Comprehensive report, along with a statement of compliance or non-compliance.

The test report shall include:

- The name and address of the testing organization and date on which the test was conducted.
- The number and year of publication of this part of ISO 14644,i.e: ISO 14644-1:2015.
- A clear identification of physical location and specific designations (a diagrammatic presentations).
- Criteria include ISO class number, the relevant occupancy state and considered particle size.
- Details of the test method used, with any special conditions relating to the test, or departures from the test methods and identification of the test instrument and its current calibration certificate.
- The test results, including particle concentration data for all sampling locations.
- If concentration of macro particles are quantified, the relevant information should be include with the test report.

5.9 Out of Specifications

- If an out of specification count is found at a location due to an identified abnormal occurrence, then that count can be discarded and note as such on the test report and a new sample taken.
- If an OOS count found at location is attributed to a technical failure of the clean room or equipment, then the cause should be identified, remedial action taken and retesting performed of the failed sampling location, the immediate surrounding location and any other locations and any other locations affected. The choice shall be clearly documented and justified.
- OOS results count shall be investigated and remedial action shall be noted in the test results.

CHAPTER 6

Good Engineering Practices in Pharmaceutical Industry

Introduction

Current Era is of GEP calls as Good engineering practices and become very challenging tool to meet new regulatory expectation. The pharmaceutical and biotech industries are highly regulated by rules that are constantly changing. It is incumbent upon engineers who are working in this area to remain up to date with Current Good Manufacturing Practices (cGMP), and to have a good understanding of the role that engineering design plays in the successful validation of a manufacturing facility. Implementation of a well-defined Good Engineering Practices (GEP) program at the initiation of a project will greatly simplify validation procedures by addressing engineering related issues that are important to the validation effort as they emerge. A good GEP program includes areas such as GMP reviews, facility layout, material and personnel flow, equipment specifications and system boundaries. This talk will focus on recent changes to the cGMP regulations that affect engineering design and validation, ISPE concepts, Maintenance qualification, Cost Reduction, simplicity and will discuss the extent to which changes can affect the manufacturing process during the design phase of the project.

Define
a Problem
Investigate
the Context
Generate
Ideas
Plan
Produce
a Solution
Evaluate

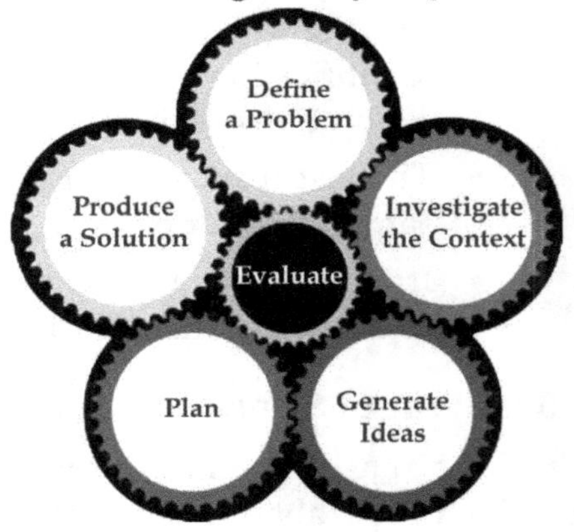

Figure 6.1 Life cycle of Good Engineering Practice.

The application of Good Manufacturing Practice to engineering is essential to ensure that a company manufactures products of the required quality. A systematic approach to Process/Facility Design is one of the foundations to a **"fit for intended use"**, compliant and cost-effective operating site. Before starting the reading the article we should have question.

What is good engineering practices?

Where we are today?

What we want to in further?

"Engineering is the systematic processes for resolve problems; Engineering is the integration of process and knowledge."

GEP is not mandated by GMP regulations. However, effective implementation and use of GEP principles improves project outcomes, team productivity, cost efficiencies, and also drives technological innovation and compliance.

6.1 Good Engineering Practice Overview

So, what is GEP? ISPE defines GEP as – "Established engineering methods and standards that are applied throughout the project lifecycle to deliver appropriate and cost-effective solutions."GEP should be applied to and provide support for specification, design, and verification activities. GEP includes specification, design, and installation activities, and should take full account of all applicable requirements, including; GxP, safety, health, environmental, ergonomic, operational, maintenance, recognized industry standards, and other statutory requirements.

Adequate provisions related to quality should be included in specification, design, procurement, and other contractual documents for engineered systems. Life-cycle documentation covering planning, specification, design, verification, installation, acceptance, and maintenance should also be produced as part of GEP.

6.2 Key Concepts in Pharmaceutical Engineering

The ISPE Good Practice Guide: Good Engineering Practice divides GEP activities into the following key concepts: Project Engineering, Common Practices, Operation and Maintenance. The guide also discusses three concepts at the core of most GEP activities: Risk Management, Cost Management and Organization and Control.

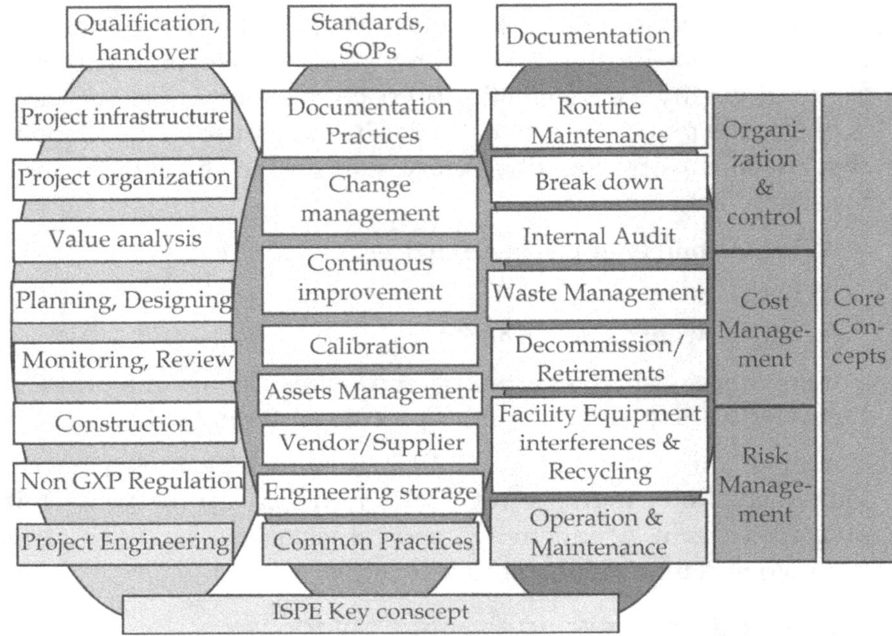

Figure 6.2 Key Concepts Good Engineering Practice.

6.3 Using Good Maintenance Practice in Good Engineering

The pharmaceutical industry should be using more condition-driven maintenance programs based upon operating data derived from predictive maintenance technologies, rather than performing maintenance on calendar basis (ISPE 2009). Figure 3 shows a matrix illustrating the relationships between Maintenance Basic, Good and Best Practices. The systems maintenance strategy is the set of criteria upon which the maintenance plans are developed. A systems maintenance strategy typically includes the following inputs

- Original equipment manufacturers recommendations;
- Experience with similar equipment;
- Review of historical data (trending);
- Process requirements;
- Risk assessment.

a. **Overall Equipment Effectiveness (OEE):** (Equipment Availability) x (Performance Efficiency) x (Rate of Quality).

b. **Types of Maintenance:** Corrective Maintenance, Preventative Maintenance and Predictive Maintenance.

c. **Levels of maintenance:** Organization maintenance level, Intermediate maintenance level and Supplier, manufacturer, depot maintenance level.

d. **Reliability Centered Maintenance:** RCM is a systematic approach to evaluate a facility's equipment and resources at high degree of facility reliability and cost-effectiveness.

e. **Availability, Reliability and Maintainability: Reliability and maintainability** are performance characteristics that combine to determine availability and can be defined as follows:

- Reliability is the time between failures under planned operating conditions. It could be described as a period of continuous, trouble-free functioning.
- Maintainability is the time needed to maintain and return failed or shut down plant elements for service.
- Availability is the fraction, ratio or percentage of time that the plant, or its subsystems is physically able to perform.

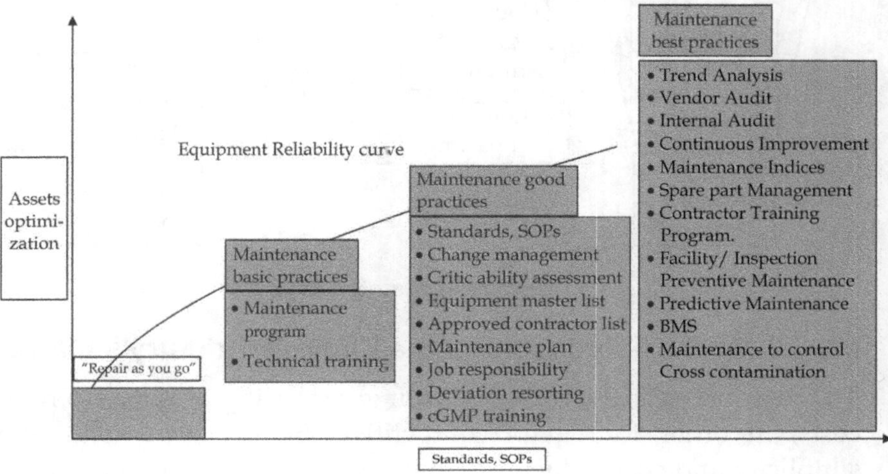

Figure 6.3 Reliability curve concept from ISPE, 2009.

6.4 Spares Management in Good Engineering Practice

Spares management includes all spares (repairable units, assemblies, and modules), repair parts (non-repairable components and piece parts), consumables (lubricants, fuels and gases), special supplies and related inventories needed to support the prime operating equipment, test and support equipment, transportation and handling equipment, training equipment, facilities and software. Excessive levels of inventory may ideally respond to the demand for spares (Operating level, Safety stock, Reorder cycle, Procurement lead time, Pipeline, Order point).

6.5 Maintenance Qualification

Maintenance qualification, provides documentary evidence of the maintenance controls in place to maintain cGMP and identifies the optimum maintenance policies required for cost-effective and efficient operations. Maintenance qualification includes Pre-screening, Impact assessment (Direct/Indirect/Non-impact). The impact assessment process is divided into two main activities. The first identifies the system boundaries and evaluates the impact of the system on the product quality. The second evaluates the criticality of the components within each direct impact system with respect to their role in assuring product quality.

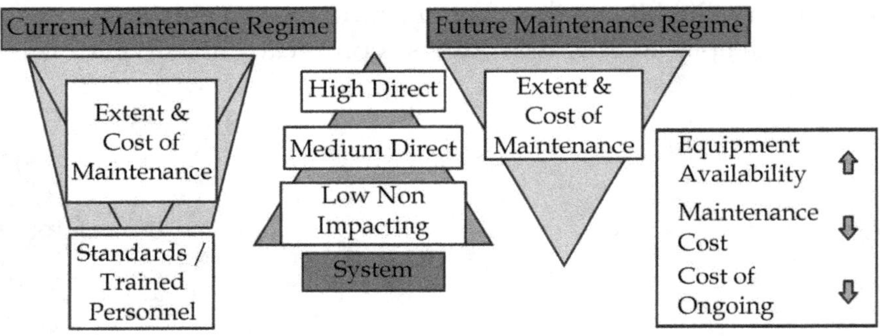

Figure 6.4 Maintenance.

6.6 Cost Cutting becomes the Pharma Industry's Mantra

The pharmaceutical industry is facing increasing pressure to reduce costs, in order to remain competitive. So everyone talks about simplicity and cost reduction. Cost cutting is rarely "good practice", however "Best Value" is very good practice. This can be achieved through a variety of ways like cost reduction through sustainable strategies, developing a streamlined and consistent global supply network, identifying global suppliers and controlling assists throughout the product development and manufacturing lifecycle.

During the cost cutting transformation, we have to identify sustainable change with the maximum long-term impact. The typically systematic approach can be adopted :

- **Aspiration-** Clear Vison.
- **Diagnostic-**Asset current and target state.
- **Specification-** Describe the impact of expected transformation.
- **Design-** Define the future go-to-market approach and operating model, starting from a clean sheet and
- **Value delivery-** Develop a transformation plan for rolling out and sustaining the necessary changes and managing the process of change itself.

6.7 Simplicity is the Ultimate Sophistication

GEP on the other hand, are simple – easy to explain, easy to test and debug and intuitive. However, simplicity should not be mistaken for "easy" or "fast.". As Steve Jobs said: **"Simple can be harder than complex and Without Complexity there is no Simplification ".** Simplifications are not easy to implement since they often require reassessing some of the core processes, methodical capability- not a traditional area of strength for pharmacos. When words "Simplicity" comes in mind, tentacles shall raise the question what will be complexity sources.

One practical way to avoid some of these complexity pitfalls is to conduct a simplicity test. The four key simplicity tests are :

- **"One sentence" test:** Can you describe every component in your architecture (or tab in your user interface or table in your schema) crisply in one sentence? As Albert Einstein said: "If you can't explain it to a 6 year old, you don't understand it yourself."
- **"What if" test:** What breaks if I don't have X? What if I don't solve this problem? What if I don't build this new component? What if I don't have this extra input box in the user interface? When it comes to systems, laziness is sometimes a good thing.
- **"Is my cost too high" test:** Complexity shows up in costs (machine, operational and integration). Know the cost of the system you are building and ask yourself if the cost is too high.

- **"Open source" test:** For every component that you build, ask yourself whether you can open-source it. Have clean and well-defined interfaces. A good test of a clean interface design is that others can easily reuse it.
- **"No, simplicity isn't easy. But taking a deliberate approach – considering the sources of complexity and asking the right questions – is a good start.**"

6.8 Measures in Good Engineering Practices

The Good Engineering Practices (GEPs) consist of proven and accepted engineering methods, procedures, and practices that provide appropriate, cost-effective, and well-documented solutions to meet user-requirements and compliance with applicable regulations. GEP underpins activities in the day-to-day operations and forward planning of a pharmaceutical business. The adoption of this methodology leads to a balance of expenditure and activity. In addition, GEP documentation can be leveraged to support verification work. To meets the current regulatory expectation more focus shall be given on three parts **Project Engineering** (Project Infrastructure, Project Organization, Value Analysis, Planning and Monitoring, Design Reviews, Handover), **Common Practices** (Standards and Procedures, Documentation Practices, Change Management and Innovation and Continuous Improvement) and **Operation and Maintenance (**Engineering Manuals and Records, Breakdown Maintenance, Internal Audit, and Equipment Decommissioning and Retirement) to strength the organization. By reviewing above documents, pharmaceutical industry will have a common understanding of the concept and principles of GEP and will be able to meet new era regulation expectations.

CHAPTER 7

Good Alarm Management Practices in Pharmaceutical Industry

Introduction

Alarm management principles, together with the ISPE, GAMP, ICH Q9, Part 11 and FDA inspection guidelines for risk management, provide a good foundation for the implementation of alarm systems in pharmaceutical manufacturing processes. This chapter gives an overview of the key principles of Alarm Management and how these can be used by the pharmaceutical industry to implement a risk based approach to alarm management to enhance productivity and implement exception reporting. A brief overview of alarm management literature and explanation of the alarm concept are provided with the aim of furthering insight and understanding.

Alarm is typical computer system or of built-in alarms to alert personnel to some out-of-limits situation or malfunction. System of alarm may be lights, buzzers, whistles, etc.

"**Alarm:** *Audible and/or Visible means of indicating to the operator an equipment malfunction, process deviation, or abnormal condition requiring a* ***timely response***" *(Figure 7.1).*

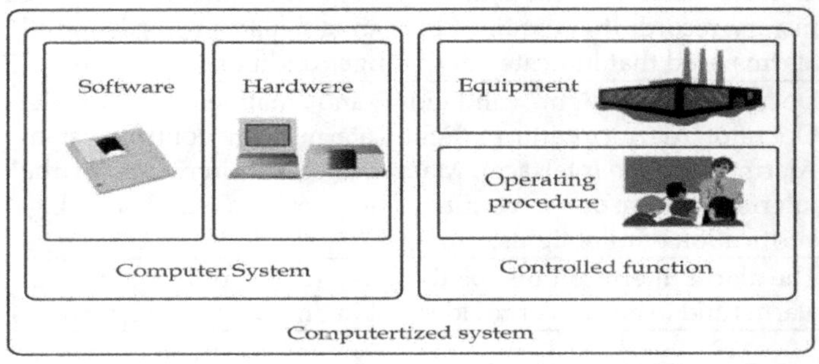

Figure 7.1 Computer system or of built-in alarms.

7.1 Key aspects of Alarm Management Program

The key aspects of alarm management can be split into four classes:

- Procedure for handling of alarm management, react to activated alarm and define effective an alarm management life cycle.
- Those that deal with the alarm handling, e.g. operator interface, design, implementation, maintenance.
- Those that deal with the alarm contents, e.g. alarm definitions, response procedures, and alarm effectiveness/performance monitoring.
- Operator act as in given table

	Operator Must Act	FYL to Operator
Abnormal	Alarm	Alert
Expected	Prompt	Message

7.2 Regulators Expectation of Alarm Management System

A. FDA and Alarming: Six expectations for alarm management as per FDA Computerized Systems in Drug Establishments (2/1983) and General Principles of Software Validation; Final Guidance for Industry and FDA Staff, January 11, 2002

S. No.	Computerized Systems in Drug Establishments Guideline	Requirement Class
1	Documentation of alarm function. The condition that initiates the alarm must be documented. Any interlocks the alarm trigger must be documented	Alarm Contents
2	Documentation of alarm parameters/thresholds and their maintenance. The alarm set-points must be documented. (Typical values are trigger point and time delay).	
3	Determination and documentation of alarm response procedure.	
4	Definition of how alarms are recorded -in batch records, logs, or automatically by the control system, and maintenance of the history record. It is required to maintain alarm records for all alarms used that indicate out of range conditions	Alarm Handling
5	Documented design, validation, and maintenance, of the Operator Alarm Interface. (lights, alarm horn, control system Alarm Manager Interface). Maintenance requirements for the interface to ensure it continues to work as validated. E.g. verification of pilot lights.	
6	The alarm interface must be designed to ensure it captures all alarms and to ensure it provides just in time access to all alarms.	Alarm Handling

B. ISA-18.2 Alarm System Management Lifecycle

- **Philosophy:** Starting point of ASM provides guidance, capability of alarm control, plan and documentation.
- **Identification: I** includes activities like P&ID reviews, process hazard reviews, layer of protection analysis and environmental permits that identify potential alarms.
- **Rationalization:** tested against the criteria documented in the alarm management to justify that it meets the requirements such as consequence, response time, Operator action, limit, priority, classification, severity define groups of alarms with similar characteristics and common requirements for training, testing, documentation, or data retention.
- **Detailed Design:** designed to meet the requirements .Alarm design includes the basic alarm design, setting parameters like the alarm designed and or off-delay time, advanced alarm design, like using process or equipment state to automatically suppress an alarm, and HMI design, displaying the alarm to the operator so that they can effectively detect, diagnose, and respond to it.

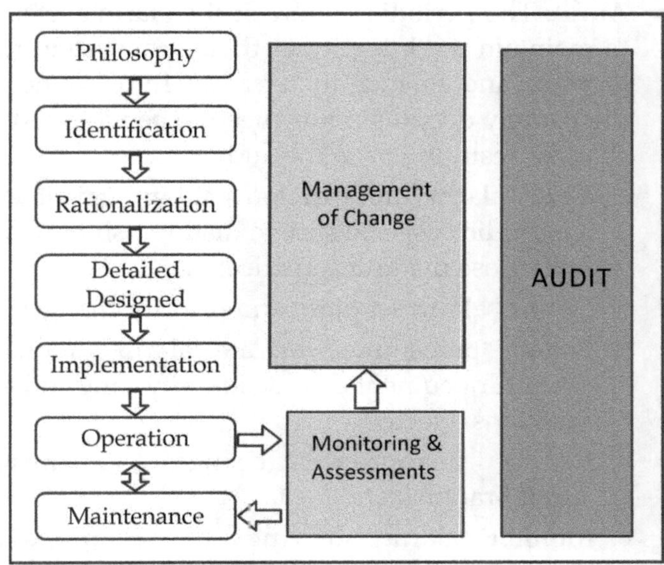

- **Implementation:** Putting the alarms into operation which includes the activities of training, testing, and commissioning.
- **Operation:** An alarm performs its function of notifying the Operator of the presence of an abnormal situation.
- **Maintenance:** In the maintenance stage the alarm does not perform its function of indicating the need for the Operator to take action as per procedure to remove an alarm from service and return an alarm to service.
- **Monitoring and Assessment:** It encompasses data gathered from the operation and maintenance stages. Assessment is the comparison of the alarm system performance against the stated performance.
- **Management of Change:** The management of change stage of the alarm lifecycle includes the activity of authorization for all changes to the alarm system, including the addition of alarms, changes to alarms, and the deletion of alarms. Once the change is approved, the modified alarm is treated as identified and processed through the stages of rationalization, detailed design and implementation again.
- **Audit:** The periodic review of the alarm system. The goal is to maintain the integrity of the alarm system throughout its lifecycle and to identify areas of improvement. The alarm philosophy document may need to be modified to reflect any changes resulting from the audit process.
  a. Verify alarm configuration settings against your design on a periodic basis. Be sure to distinguish permanent changes with those made automatically.
  b. Control alarm set point and priority changes.
  c. Follow procedures, update alarm rationalization and design documents, and identify any other alarms or functions effected.
  d. Return unapproved changes to their approved configuration state.
  e. Monitor alarm shelving and Suppression: (List of suppressed alarms, Logged comments associated with suppressed alarms, Accumulated time each alarm was suppressed and Number of times each alarm was suppressed.

7.3 Element of a Good Alarm on Risk Assessment in Pharmaceutical Industry

Alarming requirements should be collected using formal approaches such as risk assessment and element for good alarm management shall be defined.

Element of a good alarm definition include documentation of :

(a) Alarm function, the potential cause(s) that initiate the alarm. alarm interlocks.

(b) Alarm type /set point/parameters/thresholds.

(c) Escalation procedure.

(d) Allowable response time.

(e) Alarm management shall appropriately fitted to the organizational process and environmental factors.

7.4 Categorization of Alarm

Alarms can be categorized into three groups:

(a) Safety Alarms

(b) Process controls alarms

(c) Equipment alarms.

- Within each group, alarm criticality will vary according to function. All alarms directly, or indirectly, involved with the process should be individually assessed for their GMP criticality to the process. Alarm prioritization is used to indicate relative criticality between alarms. Alarm prioritization requires expert knowledge about the alarm condition and alarm response.
- Based on risk assessment ICH Q9 and ISPE guidelines, a model was developed by merging concepts from Instrumentation Management and Hazards Risk Assessment. The following three categories are suggested:

GMP Criticality	Description
1	Product Quality Critical Alarm (Exception Alarm): An alarm whose failure may have a direct impact on product quality.
2	Process / System Alarms: An alarm whose failure may affect the process or system performance but does not directly impact product quality.
3	Non- Critical Alarms: Alarms whose failure has no impact on product quality, systems or the environment.

7.5 Principle of Alarm Management System

The key Principles of Alarm Management include defining the alarms, classifying the alarms, and developing alarm response procedures. The use of GMP classification and risk assessment allows for implementation of exception reporting. Pharmaceutical companies will be well served by implementing process efficiency alarms systems to prevent production discrepancies.

CHAPTER 8

Good Computer Validation System Practices in Pharmaceutical Industry

Introduction

Computers are widely used during development and manufacturing of drugs and medical devices. Proper functioning and performance of software and computer systems play a major role in obtaining consistency, reliability and accuracy of data. Therefore, computer system validation (CSV) must be part of any good development and manufacturing practice computer systems must be validated at the level appropriate for their use and application

There are two essential parts of computerized systems:

- Infrastructure
- Applications

Validation of computer systems is not a onetime event. It starts with the planning, specification, stages of programming, testing, commissioning, documentation, operation, monitoring and modifying, product or project requirements and setting user requirement specifications and cover the vendor selection process, installation, initial operation, going use, and change control and system requirement.

For new systems validaticn starts when a user department has a need for a new computer system and thinks about how the system can solve an existing problem. For an existing system it starts when the system owner gets the task of bringing the system into a validated state. Validation ends when the system is retired and all-important quality data is successfully migrated to the new system.

Important steps in between are validation planning, defining user requirements, functional specifications, design specifications, validation during development, vendor assessment for purchased systems, installation, initial and ongoing testing and change control. In other words, computer systems must be validated during the entire life of the system.

8.1 Computer Validation Master Plan

All validation activities must be described in a validation master plan which must provide a framework for thorough and consistent validation of computer.

Computer Validation master plans must include:

Introduction with a scope of the plan, e.g., sites, systems, processes, Responsibilities by function.

Related documents, e.g., risk management plans, Products/ processes to be validated and/or qualified.

Validation approach, e.g., system life cycle approach, Risk management approach with examples of risk categories and recommended validation tasks for different categories, Vendor management, Steps for Computer System Validation with examples on type and extent of testing, for example, for IQ, OQ and PQ, Handling existing computer systems, Validation of Macros and spreadsheet calculations, Qualification of network infrastructure, Configuration management and change control procedures and templates, Back-up and recovery, Disaster recovery, Access control/ user management, Data integrity including: prevention of deletion, poor transcriptions and omission, Authorized/unauthorized changes to data and documents, Critical Alarms handling (Process Data base management system), Network system, Error handling and corrective actions, Requalification criteria, contingency planning and disaster recovery, Maintenance and support, System retirement, Training plans (e.g., system operation, compliance),Validation deliverables and other documentation and Change Control.

8.2 Computer Qualification

A. System Requirement Specifications (SRS) or User Requirement Specifications (URS)

- The vendor's specification sheets can be used as guidelines during SRS or URS.

- During SRS or URS all user department must be involved.
- The SRS or URS control documents must state the objective of a proposed computer system , the data entered , stored , the flow of data , how it interacts with other systems and procedures , the information to be produced , the limits of any variables and the operating programme and test programme.
- User requirements must have a couple of key attributes.

B. Design Qualification and Specifications

- Design qualification (DQ) defines the functional and operational specifications of the instrument and details the conscious decisions in the selection of the supplier.
- DQ must ensure that computer systems have all the necessary functions and performance criteria that will enable them to be successfully implemented for the intended application and to meet business requirements.

  a. Steps for design specification normally include:

  - Description of the task the computer system is expected to perform.
  - Description of the intended use of the system.
  - Description of the intended environment.
  - Includes network environment.
  - Preliminary selection of the system requirement specifications, functional specifications and vendor.
  - Vendor assessment.
  - Final selection of the system requirement specifications and functional specification.
  - Development and documentation of final system specifications.

C. Installation Qualification

- Installation qualification establishes that the computer system is received as designed and specified, that it is properly installed in the selected environment, and that this environment is suitable for the operation and use of the instrument. The list below includes steps as recommended before and during installation.

a. Before installation

- Obtain manufacturer's recommendations for installation site requirements.
- Check the site for the fulfillment of the manufacturer's recommendations (utilities such as electricity, water and gases and environmental conditions such as humidity, temperature, vibration level and dust).

b. During installation

- Compare computer hardware and software, as received, with purchase order (including software, accessories, spare parts).
- Check documentation for completeness (operating manuals, maintenance instructions, standard operating procedures for testing, safety and validation certificates).
- Check computer hardware and peripherals for any damage.
- Install hardware (computer, peripherals, network devices, cables).
- Install software on computer following the manufacturer's recommendation.
- Verify correct software installation, e.g., are all files accurately copies on the computer hard disk. Utilities to do this must be included in the software itself.
- Make back-up copy of software.
- Configure network devices and peripherals, e.g. printers and equipment modules.
- Identify and make a list with a description of all hardware, include drawings where appropriate, e.g., for networked data systems.
- Make a list with a description of all software installed on the computer
- Store configuration settings either electronically or on paper
- List equipment manuals and SOPs.
- Prepare an installation report.
- Both the suppliers representative and a representative of the user's form must sign off the IQ documents.

D. Operational Qualification

- Operational qualification(OQ) is the process of demonstrating that a computer system will function according to its functional specifications in the selected environment.
- During e OQ testing is done, the link between USR and DQ must be check.
- System must be tested as per vender manual or operating procedure.
- The general aspect must be also check such as power supply , temperature , magnetic disturbance.
- Training must be conducted to the user.
- Proper functioning of back-up and recovery and security functions like access control to the computer system and to data must also be tested
- Full OQ test must be performed before the system is used initially and at regular intervals.

E. Performance Qualification

- Performance Qualification (PQ) is the process of demonstrating that a system consistently performs according to a specification appropriate for its routine use i.e testing of the system with the entire application. PQ activities normally can include.
- Complete system test to proof that the application works as intended. For example for a computerized analytical system this can mean running a well characterized sample through the system and compare the results with a result previously obtained.
- Regression testing: reprocessing of data files and compare the result with previous result.
- Regular removal of temporary files
- Regular virus scan
- Auditing computer systems and Audit trails
- Security
- Back up

- Accuracy checks
- Data storage
- Printout
- Change and Configuration management

8.3 Validation Protocol/Report

- The validation protocol must be numbered, signed and dated , and must contain as a minimum the following information's.
- Objectives, Scope of coverage of the validation study.
- Validation team, their qualifications and responsibilities.
- Justification for validation.
- Risk Assessment.
- Type of validation: Prospective, concurrent, Retrospective, revalidation.
- A list of all equipment to be used with calibration, qualification, requalification and preventive maintenance details.
- Outcome of IQ , OQ for critical parameter.
- Critical parameters and their respective tolerance.
- Description of the processing steps : Challenges.
- of sampling and sampling plans.
- Statistical tools to be used in the analysis of data.
- Forms and chart to be used for documenting results.
- Non-conference (Out of Specification/Out of Trend/ Deviation).
- Change control.
- Conclusion.
- Summary.
- Approval of study.

8.4 Validation of Hardware and Software

Following aspect must be subjected to validation.

Hard ware	Soft ware
Types : • Input device • Output device • Signal converter • Central processing unit (CPU) • Distribution System • Peripheral devices	**Level :** • Machine language • Assembly language • High-level language • Application language
Key Aspect : • Location • Environment • Distance • Input device • Signal conversion • Operating system • Command overrides • Maintenance	**Software Identification:** • Language • Name • Function • Input • Output • Fix set point • Variable set point • Edits • Input manipulation • Programme overrides
Validation : • Function • Limits • Worst case • Reproducibility / Consistency • Documentation • Revalidation	**Keys Aspects :** • Software development • Software Security
	Validation : • Function • Worst case • Repeats • Documentation • Revalidation

CHAPTER 9

Good Distribution Practices — Supply Chain Integrity in Pharmaceutical Industry

Introduction

Distribution is an important activity in supply chain management of pharmaceutical medicinal products. Various people and entities are generally responsible for the products sourcing, procurement, transportation, delivery, storage, tracking and distribution of medicinal products. GDP requires adequate controls over the entire medicinal product supplier chain to protect the integrity of medicine product and help to detect adulterated drug components and drug products before entering in the supply chain.

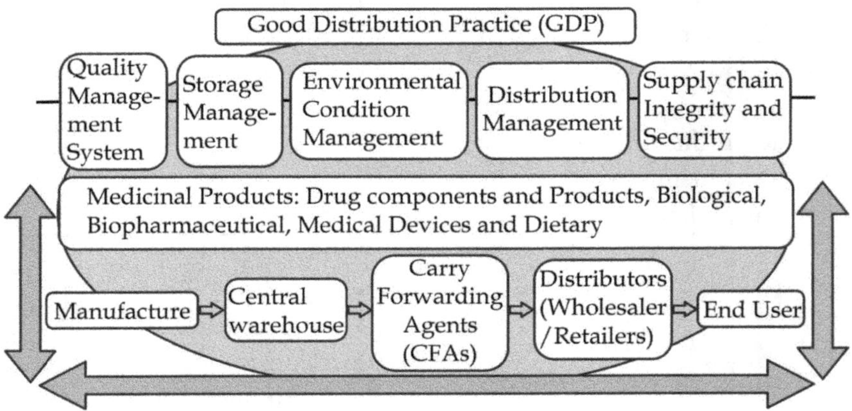

"Good Distribution Practices (GDP) is the set of standards that ensures that the quality of pharmaceuticals is maintained, without any alteration to its properties, throughout the entire cool and distribution chain, including during transportation. It is implemented by manufacturers, distributors and/or wholesalers of pharmaceutical products."

9.1 Key Components of Good Distribution Practice

A. Quality Management System

The quality system operation in distribution system must ensure that medicinal products are distributed accordance to national legislation. Authorized licence must be available for storage, distribution and transportation of medicinal products. Quality management system must ensure the right products are delivered to the right addressee within satisfactory time period at defined storage condition. Any excursion happen during the transportation of product shall be investigated and documented to impact on the product quality. Quality system must have effective mechanism to detect counterfeit medicinal product in supply chain management and recall effectively.

- **Organogram and Personnel:** Organisation must have authorized organization chart with defined duties, roles and responsibility. Personnel who are involved in the good distribution practices must be trained on receptive roles, responsibilities and approved procedure. Staff involved in these activities should have as current knowledge of suppliers, the supply chain and associated risk involved. Senior management must ensure sufficient competent personnel, equipment are available.
- **Records:** Records must be made at the time each supply chain operation is carried out in such a way that all significant activities or events are traceable. Records must be clear and readily available and retained for defined period of time as per national regulations. Records must be kept for each purchase and sale, showing the date of purchase or supply, name of the medical device, quantity received or supplied and name and address of the supplier or consignee. For transaction between different parties records must ensure the traceability's of the original and destination of product.
- **Agreement:** Witten agreement also be called as contract or quality or technical or service level agreement. An agreement is negotiated documented agreement between the drug product owner and service provider that defines the common understanding about material or service, quality specifications, roles, responsibilities, guarantees and

communication mechanisms. It can be either legally binding or an information agreement.

B. Supplier Qualification

The selection, qualification, approval and maintenance of supplier of pharmaceutical material, together with their purchase and acceptance, must be documented as part of pharmaceutical qualification. Supplier qualification is more than auditing. Supplier qualification can be seen as a risk assessment tool. It should provide an appropriate level of confidence that suppliers, vendors and contractors are able to supply consistent quality of materials, components and services in compliance with regulatory requirements. An integrated supplier qualification process should also identify and mitigate the associated risks of materials, components and services.

C. Internal Audit

Internal audits must be conducted and documented in order to monitor the implementation of the compliance with good distribution practices.

D. Storage Management system

The storage area should be sufficiently large and should have physical separate zone. The reception area should be separate from the storage and shipping/dispatch area. Records should be maintained for environment monitoring and cleaning premises. The regular checks for actual versus inventory management documents and stock rotation for first- in, first-out or first -expiration date check. Stock discrepancies shall be investigated with appropriated corrective and preventive action. Product beyond their expiry date or shelf life should be separated from usable stock. Products with broken seals, damage packaging or suspected of possible contamination must be withdrawn from saleable stock, and if not immediately destroyed, they should be kept in clearly separated area with label.

E. Environmental Condition Management

Temperatures one of the most important parameter for product storage condition which is evaluated through product stability studies. Temperature mapping of facility and vehicles plays an important role in good distribution practice. Mapping should be done based on fitness for operation during storage and transportation of medicinal product.

F. Temperature Mapping

A temperature mapping study should be designed to assess temperature uniformity and stability over the time and across a three-dimensional space. Temperature mapping should be performed in extremes whether i.e. summer and winter. Calibrated operating range data logger which are certified by NIST or other internal traceable standard should be used in temperature mapping studies. During mapping and regular monitoring should provide an alert mechanism if the preset range are breached.A three dimension temperature profile should be achieved by measuring points at not less than three dimensional planes in each directions or axis i.e. top-to-bottom, front-to-back where product will present. The temperature variability associated with mapped location and level of the thermal risk to the product should be defined in protocol. Environmental mapping a should be performed after any significant modification to the distribution system that could affect drug product temperature.

a. **Factors to be considered during Facility Temperature Mapping:** Size of the space, location of heat ventilation air conditioning system, space of heater, sun facing wall, low ceiling /roofs, geographic location of area being mapped, airflow w inside the storage location, temperature variability outside the storage location, workflow variation and movement of equipment, loading or storage pattern of product, equipment capability and standard operating procedure.

b. **Factors to be considered during Equipment (Container/trailer) Temperature Mapping:** Dedicated cargo/container/vehicles, loading and unloading procedure, route specific operation of the temperature control equipment, seasonal effected route, loading patter and transport duration.

   Excursion in environment condition shall be investigated on scientific rational and documented with the corrective and preventive action.

G. Distribution Management System

A program that covers movement, including storage and transportation of the drugs products.

- **Transportation:**

A written agreement should be available between the contract giver and contract taker include transport mode like air, road, sea, rail or a combination. Dedicated vehicles and equipment must be used for medicinal product. Where non dedicated vehicles and equipment are used ensure the quality of the medicinal product will not compromised. Vehicles cleanliness should be check and record before loading or unloading of medicinal products.

9.2 Counterfeit

Counterfeit products discovered in the distribution network must be immediately brought to the attention of the competent authority as well as the manufacturer of the genuine product. Such products have to be clearly identified and put under quarantine to prevent further distribution or sale. Upon confirmation of the product being counterfeit a formal decision should be taken on its disposal, ensuring that it does not re-enter the market and the decision should be recorded.

9.3 Supply Chain Integrity and Security

Supply chain is used to control the storage and distribution lifecycle of the a product to the end user. Supply chain must be transparent and traceability with documentation at each and very receipt and dispatch of medicinal product. Periodic verification of supply chain and security should be performed to assess the risk in medicinal product distribution. Supply chain and security consist of:

- **Product identification:**

  Manufacturers and repackagers to put a unique product identifier on certain prescription drug packages, for example, using a bar code that can be easily read electronically.

- **Product tracing:**

  Manufacturers, wholesaler drug distributors, repackagers, and many dispensers in the drug supply chain to provide information about a drug and who handled it each time it is sold in the market.

- **Product verification:**

  Manufacturers, wholesaler drug distributors, repackagers, and many dispensers to establish systems and processes to be able to verify the product identifier on certain prescription drug packages.

- **Detection and response:**

  Manufacturers, wholesaler drug distributors, repackagers, and many dispensers to quarantine and promptly investigate a drug that has been identified as suspect, meaning that it may be counterfeit, unapproved, or potentially dangerous.

- **Notification:**

  Manufacturers, wholesaler drug distributors, repackagers, and many dispensers to establish systems and processes to notify regulator and other stakeholders if an illegitimate drug is found.

- **Wholesaler licensing:**

  Wholesale drug distributors to report their licensing status and contact information to regulators. This information will then be made available in a public database.

- **Third-party logistics provider licensing:**

  Third-party logistic providers, those who provide storage and logistical operations related to drug distribution, to obtain a state or federal license

9.4 Category of Supply Chain Integrity and Security

Supply chain integrity and security mainly falls in following five category:

- **Cargo management:**

  Protecting cargos during all steps of manufacturing, shipping and transport processes.

- **Facility management:**

  Security of the facilities where goods are manufactured, stored and handled.

- **Information management:**

  Protecting critical business data and exploiting information as tool for detecting illegal activities and preventing security breaches.

- **Human resource management:**

  Trustworthiness and security awareness of all personnel with physical or virtual access to the supply chains.

- **Company management systems:**

  Building security into internal and external organizational structures and company management systems including supplier, partners and client management processes.

  Overall the Drug Supply Chain Security is the Collaboration of Good manufacturing practices, Good distribution practices, Good import/export practices, Clinical/retail pharmacy practices, Product security, Detection technology, Internet sales, Track and trace systems, Surveillance and monitoring and Single points of contact.

CHAPTER 10

Good Data Management System in Pharmaceutical Industry

Introduction

In recent years there has been a significant increase in the number and types of data integrity issues that have been cited in regulatory inspections. Regulatory focus on the integrity of electronic and paper-based data has increased sharply. Data integrity issues have been increasing to become one of the most important GMP issues. This increase has led to red flags and triggering a more intensive investigation. Data integrity and Data governance system is fundamental in a pharmaceutical quality system which ensures that medicines are of the required quality. Systems should be designed in a way that encourages compliance with the Principles of data integrity.

"Confidence in the quality and the data generated integrity is a fundamental of Data reliability."

Before starting discussion, terms need to be understand such as:

- **Data:** Facts, figures and statistics collected together for reference or analysis(*ALCOA)*
- **Data Governance:** The sum total of arrangements to ensure that data, irrespective of the format in which it is generated, is recorded, processed, retained and used to ensure a complete, consistent and accurate record throughout the data lifecycle.

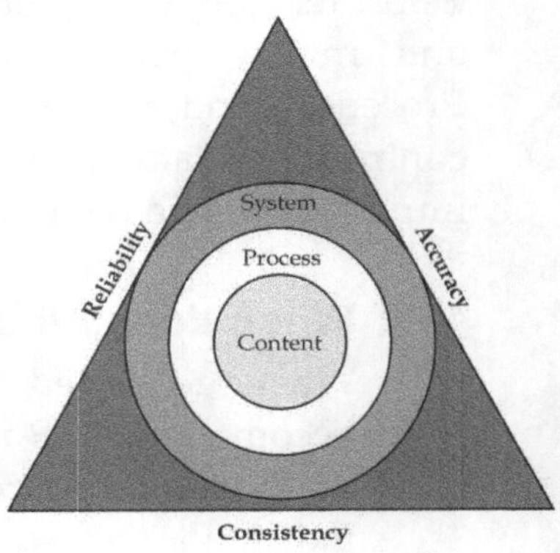

- **Data Integrity:** The extent to which all data are complete, consistent and accurate throughout the Data lifecycle.

- **Data Lifecycle:** All phases in the life of the data (including raw data) from initial generation and recording through processing (including transformation or migration), use, data retention, archive / retrieval and destruction.
- **ALCOA:** Data to be **A**ttributable, **L**egible, **C**ontemporaneous, **O**riginal, and **A**ccurate.

A L C O A	Attributable	Who acquired the data or performed an action and when?
	Legible	Can you read the data?
	Contemporaneous	Documented at the time of the activity
	Original/Reliable	Written printout or observation or a certified copy thereof
	Accurate	No errors or editing without documented amendments

10.1 Regulatory Expectations

Data integrity applies to all pharmaceutical quality management system and apply equally to manual (paper) and electronic data. Data integrity applies to all an organization with respect to people, systems and facilities to ensure data is complete consistent and accurate in all its forms, i.e. paper and electronic. Periodic data verification should done and documented for its correctness, accurate legibility and exiting controls are working fine. Regulators expects industry should balance data risk with other quality and compliance priorities. Risk to data integrity should communicate the senior management and action should be taken on the prioritization .Short term and long term action plan with measure shall be traced and review periodically for its effectiveness and completion. Procedure and system controls should be available to review and control the data integrity. Periodic personnel training plays an important role in data integrity.

10.2 When does Electronic Data become a CGMP Record?

- When generated to satisfy a CGMP requirement, all data become a CGMP record which cannot be modified and static or dynamic nature of the original records. Static is used to indicate a fixed-data document such as a paper record or an electronic image, and dynamic means that the record format allows interaction between the user and the record content.

- Data integrity requirements applicable to:
- API and FP manufacturers, including contract manufacturing
- Testing units, including contract laboratories.
- Outsourced GMP activities such as equipment qualification and calibration.

10.3 CIA or AIC Triangle

CIA triangle or *AIC* triangle (availability, integrity and Confidentiality) is a model designed to guide policies for information security within an Organization. The elements of the triangle are considered the three most crucial components of data security: **Confidentiality** - set of rules that limits access to information, **Integrity** - assurance that the information is trustworthy and accurate, and **Availability**- A guarantee of reliable access to the information by authorized people.

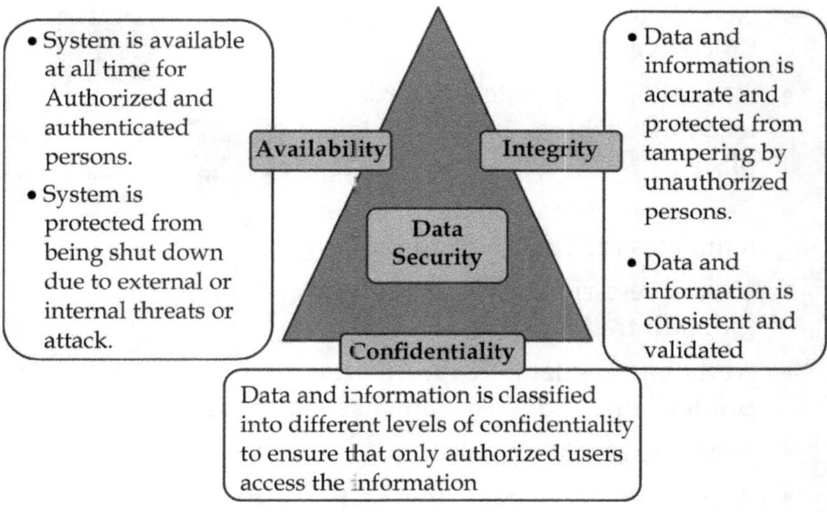

10.4 The Data Governance System

The data governance system should be integral to the pharmaceutical quality system and shall be controlled organizational (procedural) and technically (electronically).The data information may be qualitative or quantitative or numerical values or text or images or drawings or audio or video records or it can come from a variety of sources. The key is that the data must be responsibly managed and secure. Data management encompasses several different tasks such as **6 D concept module system:** Data selection, Data analysis, Data handling, Data reporting, Data Issuance and **Data ownership.**

Two other important aspects of data governance system include the validated state of a process or a computerized system (ensuring accuracy of generated or recorded data), and the management of critical authorizations (protection of data to avoid integrity breaches during operation).

Risk management approach can be applied based on Data criticality and its risk.

10.5 Designing Systems to Assure Data Quality and Integrity

Systems should be designed in a way that encourages compliance with the ***Principles of data integrity***. Examples include:

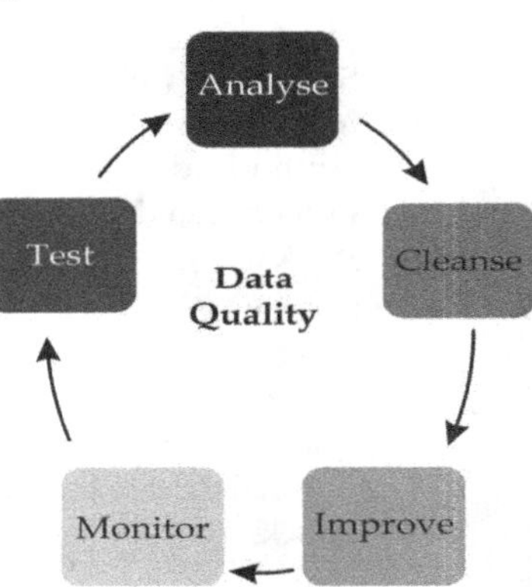

- Access to clocks for recording timed events
- Accessibility of batch records at locations where activities take place
- Control over blank paper templates for data recording ,
- User access rights which prevent (or audit trail) data
- Automated data capture or printers attached to equipment such as balances
- Access to sampling points
- Access to raw data for staff performing data checking activities.

10.6 Triggers of Data Integrity Loss

Triggers of data integrity loss involves attacks on data integrity which can be intentional and non-intentional, during the data life cycle. Triggers of data integrity loss may due to changes to access permissions and privileges, Inability to track the use of privileged passwords, Passwords shared, End-user error that impacts production data, Vulnerable code-in applications, Weak or immature change control and accreditation processes, Misconfiguration of security devices and software, Incorrectly or incompletely applied patches, Unauthorized devices and Unauthorized applications connected to the corporate network, Inadequate or not applied segregation of duties ,Processing and/or deriving data Deleting, removing and destroying data, replicating and distributing data, Archiving and recalling data ,Backing up and restoring data

10.7 Data Integrity Metrics

Data integrity matrix framework is based on three complementary approaches.

- ***First***: looks at specific known and uses attacks to analyze their probability,
- ***Second***: addresses this limitation by applying cryptographic "provable security" results
- ***Third***: approach building information system components by establishing, implementing, measuring, and maintaining and review data integrity across an organization

10.8 Measures of Good Data Management System

The message for data integrity is clear. It's not a new concept; it's about getting back to the roots of training all staff on the importance of data integrity in cGMP documentation and honesty. It is critical to ensure employees understand the accountability and traceability requirements for retention of raw data and the consequences of data manipulation. Training operators and analysts to document the performance of a task by recording what happened at the time it occurs, including information about the person who performed it along with clearly documenting and investigating deviations, is vital for patient safety and product efficacy. This is achievable by providing the training and creating a company culture that promotes and rewards ethical behavior as a core value from top to bottom of an organization.

CHAPTER 11

Quality Agreements in Pharmaceutical Industry

Introduction

Quality agreement is legally binded and mutual negotiation between two parties that is Contract Giver and Contract Acceptor. It define, in a formalized manner, clear role and responsibilities relative to quality tasks to assure the manufacture and supply of safe materials

"A quality agreement is a comprehensive written agreement between parties involved in the contract manufacturing of drugs that defines and establishes each party's manufacturing activities in terms of how each will comply with CGMP."

Quality agreements is based on cGMP principles by defining, establishing, and documenting their activities in drug manufacturing operations, including processing, packing, holding, labeling operations, testing, and quality control operations. Quality Agreement should not cover general business terms and conditions such as confidentiality, pricing or cost issues, delivery terms, or limits on liability or damages.

11.1 Elements of a Quality Agreement

- Quality agreements should made in formalized documents with clear well-written language. It define key roles and responsibilities communication mode, services, expectations, and approval of varies activities of both parties. Element of a Quality agreement are as follows, but not limited to;
- ***Purpose/Scope***: To cover the nature of the contract manufacturing services to be provided.

- *Definitions* : To ensure that the owner and contract facility agree on precise meaning of terms in the quality agreement.
- *Resolution of disagreements*: To explain how the parties will resolve disagreements about product quality issues or other problems.
- *Manufacturing activities*: To document quality unit and other activities associated with manufacturing processes as well as control of changes to manufacturing processes.
- Life cycle of, and revisions to, the quality agreement.

11.2 Activities in Quality Agreements

a. **Quality unit:**

Following activities are involved;

- Quality activity to ensure the product meets cGMP activities.
- Approving, rejection and dispatches of product.
- Communication between each other.
- Audits, inspections, and communication of findings.
- Communicating inspection observations and findings.

b. **Facilities and equipment:**

Following activities are involved;

- Facility as per cGMP.
- Qualification, Validation, Calibration, Preventive maintenance.
- Technology and automated control systems, environmental monitoring and room classification, utilities, and any other equipment and facilities.
- It should indicate how the parties will communicate information about preventing cross-contamination and maintaining traceability when a contract facility processes drugs for multiple owners.

c. **Materials management:**

Following activities are involved;

- Auditing, qualifying, and monitoring component suppliers.
- Sampling and testing in compliance with CGMP.

- Inventory management, including labeling, label printing, inventory reconciliation, and product status identification.
- Facility prevent mix-ups and cross-contamination.
- Define responsibility for physical control of materials at different points in the manufacturing process.
- Each party's roles in storage and transport.
- Each party's roles in Environmental conditional monitoring during storage and transport.

d. **Product-specific considerations:**

Following activities are involved;

- Product/component specifications.
- Defined manufacturing operations, including batch numbering processes.
- Responsibilities for expiration/retest dating, storage and shipment, and lot disposition.
- Responsibilities for process validation, including design, qualification, and ongoing verification and monitoring.
- Provisions to allow owner personnel access to the contract facility when appropriate.
- Product knowledge, Product development report technology transfer.

e. **Laboratory controls:**

Following activities are involved;

- Procedures delineating controls over sampling and testing samples.
- Protocols and procedures for communicating all laboratory test results conducted by contract facilities to the owner for evaluation and consideration in final product disposition decisions.
- Procedures to verify that both owner and contract facilities accurately transfer development, qualification, and validation methods when an owner uses a contract facility for laboratory testing.
- Routine auditing procedures to ensure that a contract facility's laboratory equipment is qualified, calibrated, and maintained in a controlled state in accordance with CGMP.

- Designation of responsibility for investigating deviations, discrepancies, failures, out-of-specification results and out-of-trend results in the laboratory, and for sharing reports of such investigations.

f. **Documentation:**

Following activities are involved;

- Review and approval of documents.
- Changes made to standard operating procedures, manufacturing records, specifications, laboratory records, validation documentation, investigation records, annual reports, and other documents related to products or services provided by the contract facility.
- Roles in making and maintaining original documents or true copies in accordance with CGMP.
- Records readily available during audit, inspection or whenever required.
- Electronic records: storage, periodic review and retrieval.
- Record-keeping time frames.

CHAPTER 12

Change Control Management and its Applications

Introduction

Change control is important an element of pharmaceutical Quality Management system and is closely interwoven with regulatory compliance. The change control system provides transparency and a structured approach towards end- to end changes. Change control system provides checks and balances in the quality system by initiating, reviewing, approving, distribution, tracking and storing change history throughout the life cycle. It also links to other quality and regulatory processes such as corrective and preventive action (CAPA) and product registration tracking.

The scope of the change control program must be border than change control, which typically applied to one change at a time. The change control management should have a broad set of possibilities view on changes to product formulation or design, upgrades to facilities, utilities, equipment and computer systems, manufacturing instructions, SOPs, test methods and specifications, any new raw materials as well as any changes in policy.

12.1 Benefits of Change Control System

- Structured and consistent approach towards managing changes.
- Documenting the details of change.
- Routing of change requests to appropriate individuals/team for approvals.
- Documentation of change approvals and implementation.
- Maintenance of change history and easy retrieval of information.

- Tracking changes effectively and providing an audit trail.
- Demonstrate compliance to regulations.
- The change management system should include the following, as appropriate for the stage of the lifecycle.

12.2 ICH Q8 and ICH Q9 to Change Management in ICH Q10

Change Management: A systematic approach to proposing, evaluating, approving, and implementing and reviewing changes. (ICH Q10).

The change management system should include the following:

- Quality risk management should be utilized to evaluate proposed changes;
- The level of effort and formality of the evaluation should be commensurate with the level of risk;
- Proposed changes should be evaluated relative to the marketing authorization, including current product and process understanding and/or design space, where established;
- Expert teams, with appropriate expertise and knowledge, should evaluate proposed changes;
- An evaluation of the change should be undertaken after implementation to confirm the change objectives were achieved.

12.3 Steps involved in Change Control Management

- Login of Change Control and description.
- Description of Changes: Reason for change, Proposed changes, justification for change.
- Type of Change Control : Facility /System/ Documentation / Product.
- Assigning the task to Cross function teams.
- Risk Analysis and Impact Assessment.
- Change control Categorization Major / Minor Change Control
- Approval of Change control :
- Implementation of Change Control.

- Results/ Effectiveness of the Actions.
- Verification and closure.

12.4 E-Change Control System

Electronic change control management helps to managing all change control processes in a centralized and harmonized manner. It helps in proper coordination across stakeholders through automated workflows and alerts if any timelines are crossed. It increases operational transparency through automated alerts, summary dashboard functionality, and extensive reporting capabilities. It also increases accountability though assignments, process step sign-offs, and automated audit trails. Electronic change control processes increase compliance, enable companies to reduce costs, liability and patient risk.

CHAPTER 13

Technology Transfer of Pharmaceutical Product

Introduction

Transfer of technology is defined as a logical procedure that controls the transfer of an essential process together with its documentation and professional expertise to a site capable of reproducing the process and its support functions to a predetermined level of performance

Transfer of technology requires a planned approach using trained and knowledgeable personnel working staff within a robust quality system, with documentation of data covering all aspects of production and quality control.

In order for the transfer to be successful, the following requirements should be ensure by organization and management:

- The facilities and equipment at the sending unit (SU) and receiving unit (RU) should be equivalent.
- Adequate trained staff should be available at the RU.
- Well Documentation: SOP, protocol and reports, specification, critical process parameters and supportive data should be transferred from the SU to the RU.
- A time frame should be defined for the transfer project.
- Regulatory requirement should be taken of SU and RU should be taken into the consideration.

13.1 Different Types of Technology Transfer

a. Technology Transfer from R&D to Production.

b. Technology Transfer from one unit to other unit.

c. Technology Transfer from one location to other location.

d. During the technology transfer following areas at the sending unit (SU) and receiving unit (RU) should be consider:

- The technology transfer should be established at the outset whether the intention is to perform single batch manufacturer, continuous production or campaigns and whether the RU can accommodate the intended production capacity.
- The SU should provide the drug master file (DMF) for active and inactive material.
- Depending upon the type of dosage form, the SU should provide relevant information on physical properties of material to RU.
- Process information: The SU should provide a detail history of process development, characterization of the product including qualitative and qualitative composition, physical description, method of manufacture, in-process control, specification packaging components and configurations, safety and handling procedure.
- The SU should provide Cleaning and Packaging procedure to RU.
- The SU should provide analytical methods to test the pharmaceutical product or material to RU.
- The SU should provide necessary validation documentation for the process and its support function.
- The SU should asses the suitability and degree of preparedness of the RU before transfer in terms of premises, equipment and services support (e.g Purchasing and inventory control mechanisms, quality control procedures, documentation, computer validation, site validation, equipment qualification, waste management etc).
- The SU and the RU should jointly implement training programme specific to the product, process or to be transferred, e.g. analytical methods or equipment usage and assess training outcomes.
- The SU and the RU should jointly document the execution of the transfer protocol in a transfer report.

13.2 Technology Transfer Protocol and Report

Contents of technology transfer protocol are :

- *Product Name*: Generic or/and Brand name with strength.
- Objective and Scope.
- Key person name of Sender and Receiving Unit.
- Responsibility of Sender Unit and Receiving Unit.
- Comparison of Materials/Methods/Equipment/Facilities of Sender and Receiving Unit.
- Identification of critical control parameters.
- Experimental design and acceptance criteria for analysis for analytical methods.
- Information on trial production batches, qualification batches and process validation.
- Change Control for any process deviations encountered, Assessment of End-Product.
- Reference samples of active ingredients, intermediates and Finished products.
- Conclusion.

CHAPTER 14

Pharmaceutical Annual Product Quality Review

Introduction

Annual product quality review is also called as APQR. It an effective tool to verify the consistency of existing process, the appropriateness of current specifications for both starting material and finished product to highlight any trends and to identify product and process improvement. It is regular periodic or rolling quality reviews of medical products. The APQR capture a border view of product data, capturing trends and helps to determine the need for revalidation and changes if any and help can be considered part of the continuous improvement process. The purpose of an APR or PQR is not only to assess the quality of products, processes and systems, but also to offer the possibility of checking the current state of the marketing authorization with regard to conformity of the following to the data submitted:

14.1 Importance of Annual Product Quality Review

- Trends help to determine the defect regarding product stability.
- Helps needs of revalidation.
- It verifies the consistency of the existing manufacturing processes.
- It determines the quality and process defects of the products.
- It determines the defects and possible improvements of the methods and process.
- Trend of yield, analytical results, manufacturing parameters of the product are also highlighted.

- It reviews the quality of the raw material and packaging material which is used for the product.
- Mainly it indicates the quality of material.
- To determine the consistency of the quality of the product the in-process parameters and the finished product results are reviewed.
- Quantity of the final product is reviewed by trending the yield of every batch.

14.2 Contents of APQR

- Scope.
- Product information: Generic or Brand name, Therapeutic category, Shelf life, Product code, Batch manufactured formula number, Manufacturing License number, Marketing Authorization number.
- Information: Batch Size, Number of Batches manufactured, Number of Work in Progress, Batches Packed with Pack size.
- Review Period and Unique APQR number.
- A review of Starting material: Raw material, Intermediates, Key stating Material and Packing Materials with vendor qualification details critical.
- Review of critical in-process control, test results and Yield;
- Review of Validations: Process validation, Cleaning Validation.
- Review of different pack size.
- Review of Qualification: Equipment's and Utilities.
- Review of Out of Specification (Valid and In-Valid OOS).
- Review of Out of Trend.
- Review of Stability data.
- Review of reserve sample.
- Review of Complaints.
- Review of Recall or Returns or Salvage goods.
- Review of Change controls (any changes carried out to the processes or analytical methods or Art work changed).
- Review of Technical or GMP Agreement.

- Review of Marketing Authorization.
- Review of Previous APR.
- Conclusions and Recommendations.
- Approval.

14.3 Data Trend and Analyzation

The data should be trended and analyzed to determine if (i) the process is in control; and (ii) the process is capable. Control limits should be established through trending. The appropriateness of current specifications for both starting materials and finished product should also be determined. In addition, it is important to highlight any trends observed and to identify product and process improvements. Improvement plans and actions should be initiated and taken if the process is found to be out of control or has low capability indices.

The data may be analyzed using the following techniques:

Control Chart

- Control charts (example: X-bar charts, R-charts and Moving Range charts etc.) can be used to determine upper and lower control limits, and identify trends ,so that appropriate actions may be taken before out-of specification occurs.

Process Capability Study

- Processcapability indices are used to measure how well the data fits into the specification limits. Frequently used process capability indices include Cp and Cpk. Cp is used to evaluate the variation of the process, and Cpk is used to evaluate the centering of the process. It is important for manufacturers to calculate and analyse the values of Cp and Cpk for their processes and understand the interpretation of such data. It is recommended that the Cp / Cpk values be targeted at 1.33 or above. Process capability studies assist manufacturers in determining if the specifications limits set are appropriate, and also to highlight processes that are not capable. Manufacturers would then be required to take necessary improvement plans/actions.

CHAPTER 15

Statistical Tools for Pharmaceutical Industry

Introduction

Statistics are critical to the pharmaceutical industry, from clinical operations through manufacturing. However, clinical and manufacturing statistics represent entirely different worlds. According to current requirement of regulatory expectation and warning letter, extensive statistical knowledge is very important. Without extensive statistical knowledge, the requirements for GMP can be mysterious and intimidating. Qualitative or Quantitative statistical tool can be used for analysed of data. Statistical tool should not be only Data mining or data pooing .The usage of correct statistical tools at the right time is very important to understand quality level. This chapter consist of fundamental concepts in statistical analysis, concept of six sigma and lean manufacturing, statistical tools: measurement system analysis, control chart, capability, acceptance sampling, stability analysis, frequency, distributions, process capability, qualitative and quantitative analysis, patterns and trends.

Statistics is concerned with scientific methods for collecting, organizing, summarizing, presenting, and analysing data, as well as drawing valid conclusions and making reasonable decisions on the basis of such analysis. Statistics is a simple method of extracting information from what often seems at first glance to be a mass of random numbers.

"Measures of central tendency and dispersion are the two most fundamental concepts in statistical analysis."

- **MEASURES OF CENTRAL TENDENCY:** Most frequency distributions exhibit a 'central tendency' i.e., a shape such that the bulk of the observations pile up in the area between the two extremes. Central tendency is one of the most fundamental concepts in all statistical analysis. There are three principal measures of central tendency:

a. **Mean**-average of the total of the sample values.
b. **Median**-the middle value (midpoint) of a data, and
c. **Mode**-the value or number that occurs most frequently in a data set.

DISPERSION: Dispersion is the variation in the spread of data about the mean. Dispersion is also referred to as variation, spread, and scatter. A measure of dispersion is the second of the two most fundamental measures of all statistical analyses. Data are always scattered around the zone of central tendency, and the extent of this scatter is called dispersion or variation. There are several measures of dispersion: **range-**difference between the maximum and minimum values in an observed data set, **standard deviation-** measures the extent of dispersion around the zone of central tendency, and **coefficient of variation**-final measure of dispersion: the guaranteed existence of a difference between any two items or observations. Concept of variation states that no two observed items will ever be identical.

15.1 Concept of Six Sigma and Lean Manufacturing

- **Six Sigma:**

  A unique approach to improve the quality which was developed and implanted by Motorola. Six sigma is a statistical methodology that focuses on the reducing variation and defects, and mistake-proofing a process. Six sigma data-driven approach to process improvements is divided into five phase: **Define, Measure, Analyse, Improve and control.**

- **Lean Manufacturing:**

  Lean manufacturing is a strategy for achieving the shortest possible cycle time by eliminating waste and unnecessary process steps, reducing inventory, reducing product development time and increasing customer responsiveness while providing high quality product. **Lean manufacturing dependents on five basic principle:** Values-from customer perspective, Value steam-A series of activity, Flow-getting product to move without stopping, Pull-supplying for customer and Perfection-this is an iterative cycle of continuous improvement.

15.2 Common Statistical Tools Pharmaceutical Industry can use to Meet Regulatory Requirements

- **Measurement System Analysis (MSA):**

  An experimental and mathematical method of determining how much the variation within the measurement process contributes to overall process variability. **There are five parameters to investigate in an MSA:** Accuracy, Repeatability, Reproducibility, Stability and Adequate Resolution.

  DOE can be conducted by: Conduct an experiment where different people / machines measure, plot the data, analyse the data. Use statistical techniques such as Analysis of Variance and improve the measurement process, if necessary.

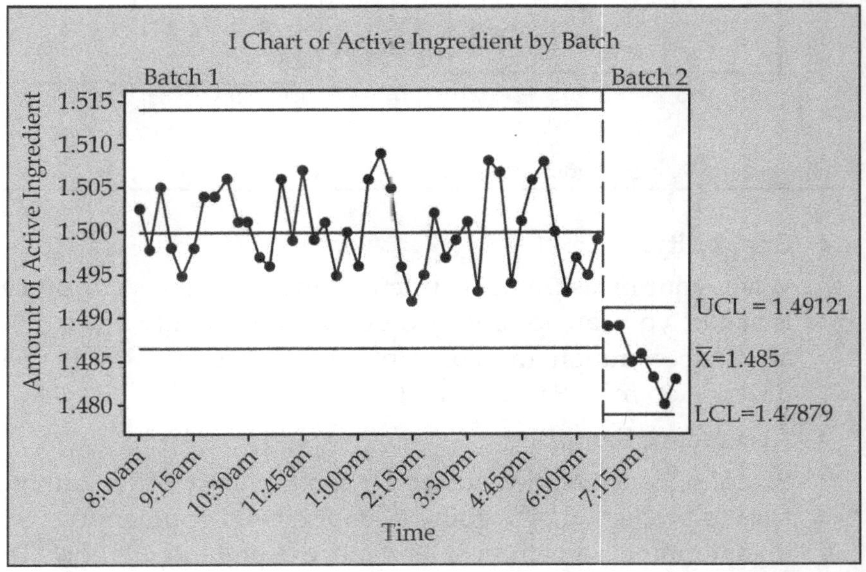

- **Control Chart:**

  The control chart is a graph used to study how a process changes over time. Data are plotted in time order. A control chart always has a central line for the average, an upper line for the upper control limit and a lower line for the lower control limit. These lines are determined from historical data.

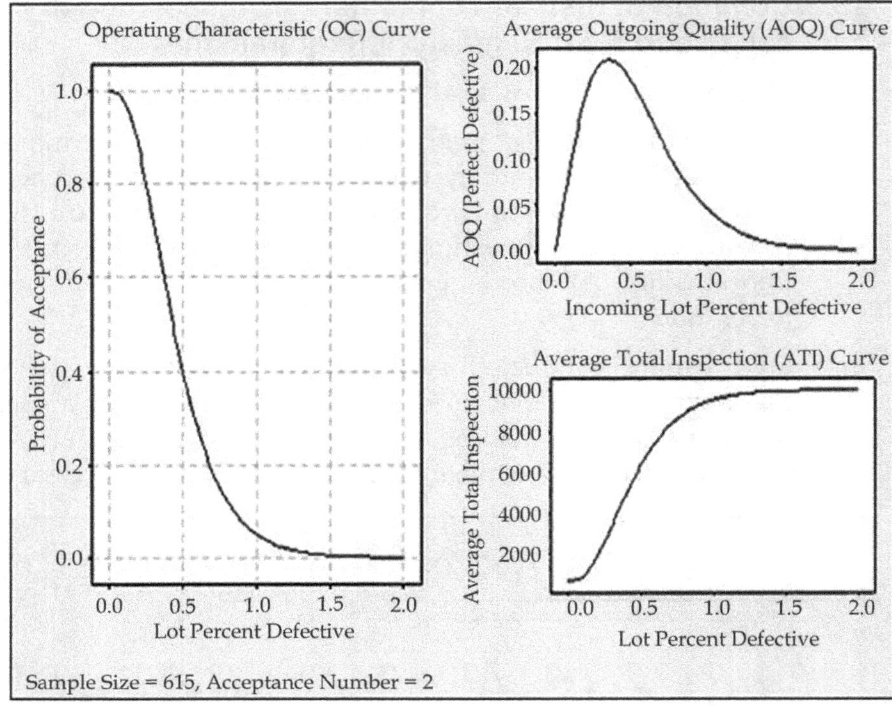

- **Capability:**

  When your measurement system is adequate and your process is stable, you can accurately describe your quality level. There are four common measures of process quality level. (Brief description refer Process capability section).

- **Acceptance Sampling:**

  Sampling is a complex subject. It can be divided into analytic: tries to predict what is going to happen and enumerative: tries to determine something about an existing population. Two statistics acceptance sampling plans used in industry: Average outgoing quality (AOQ): Represents the defect rate after implementing a sampling plan and Average total inspection (ATI): represents the average number of pieces that you inspect.

- **Stability Analysis:**

  Stability analysis evaluates how your product degrades over time during shipment and storage. The data collection for stability involves taking samples from at least three batches, storing the samples at the manufacturing facility, and measuring samples from each batch at regular time intervals.

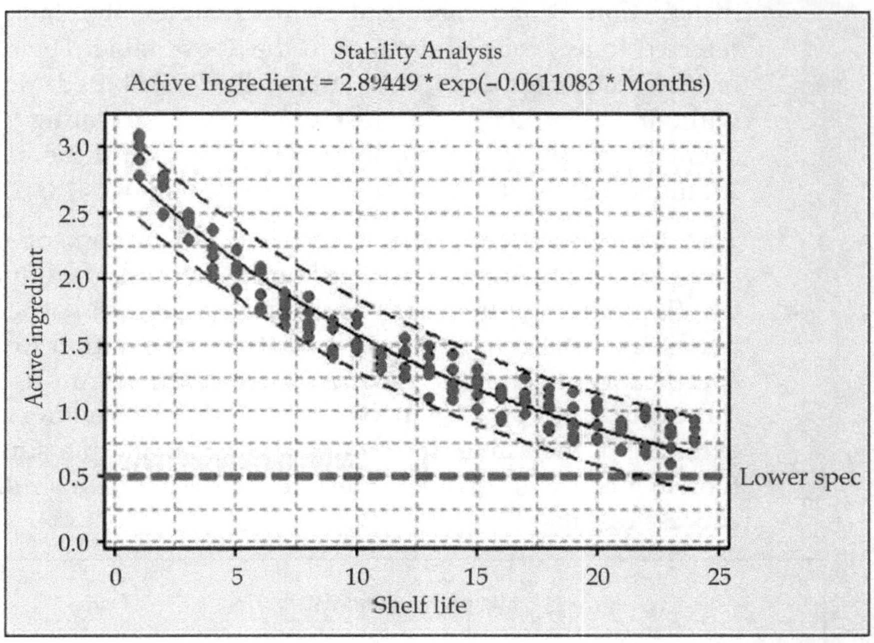

15.3 Other Statistical Tools used in Pharmaceutical Industry

a. Frequency Distributions:

Class Boundaries	Mid-point	Frequency	Cumulative frequency
14.5-15.4	15	2	2
15.5-16.4	16	9	11
16.5-17.4	17	24	35
17.5-18.4	**18**	29	64
18.5-19.4	19	25	89
19.5-20.4	20	8	97
20.5-21.4	21	3	100

A **frequency** distribution is a tool for presenting data in a form **that** clearly demonstrates the relative frequency of the occurrence of values as well as the central tendency and dispersion of the data. Raw data are divided into classes to determine the number of values in a class or class frequency. The data are arranged by classes, with the corresponding frequencies in a table called a frequency distribution. When organized in this manner, the data are referred to as grouped data, as in the above table. The data in this table appear to be normally distributed. Even without constructing a histogram or calculating the average, the values appear to be centered around the value 18. In fact, the arithmetic average of these values is 18.02.

The histogram provides a graphic illustration of the dispersion of the data. Histogram may be used to compare the distribution of the data to specification limits in order to determine where the process is centered in relation to the specification tolerances. Frequency distributions are useful for evaluating process performance and presenting the evidence of their analysis. Not only is a histogram a simple tool to use, it is also an effective method of illustrating process results.

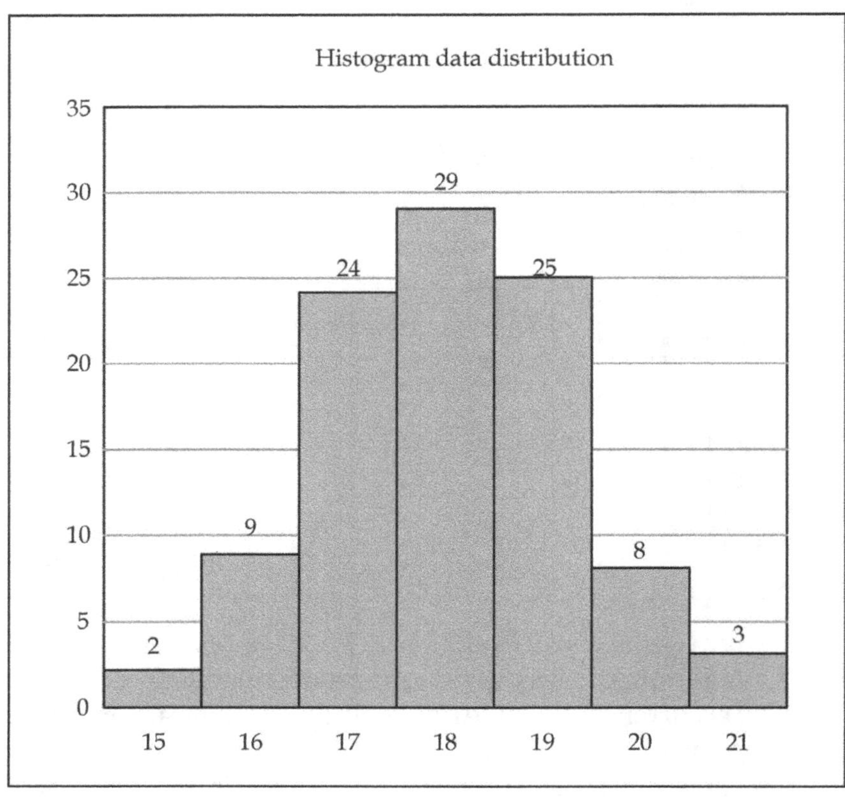

b. Process Capability (PC):

Process capability provides a quantified prediction of the adequacy of a process. It also measures the capability of a process to produce products that meet specifications by measuring the inherent uniformity of the process.

PC indices numerically express the relationship between the distribution and the specification limits. A process is in a state of statistical control when the plotted data points are within the calculated UCL and LCL almost all the time (such as 99.73 percent) and the data do not display a particular form that would indicate an out-of-control condition or instability. A process is capable when the distribution of individual piece data is within or equal to the upper specification limit (USL) and the lower specification limit (LSL).

A process capability index expresses a numerical relationship between the process variability and the specification limits. The indices currently used are C_r, C_p, C_{pk} and C_{pm}.

- C_r *and* C_p are ratios of the specification tolerance (USL – LSL) to the process spread (6σ). The difference between them is that Cp.

  $C_p = \frac{USL - LSL}{6\sigma}$ is the reciprocal of Cr $C_p = \frac{6\sigma}{USL - LSL}$

  fthe UCL and the LCL are superimposed on the USL and the LSL, the Cp would equal 1. This assumes that the mean of the process is exactly centered within the specification limits. If the control limits fall outside the specification limits, the value of Cp would be less than 1.

- C_{pk} is a method of measuring process capability when the mean of the process is not centered with regard to the specification limits.

  $$C_{pk} = \text{Min}\left[\frac{USL - X}{3\sigma}, \frac{X - LSL}{3\sigma}\right]$$

- A C_{pk} of 1 or greater means that the process is capable at a level of at least 99.73 percent conforming, which is the limit associated with an X– and an R chart. It is extremely important when using these capability indices that the process be in control because the theory is based entirely on a normal distribution. If the distribution is not normal, the indices are meaningless

- *Cpm* takes into account variation between the process average and a target value.

$$C_{pm} = \text{Min}\left[\frac{\text{USL} - \text{LSL}}{6/\sigma^2 + \left(X - \mu^2\right)}\right]$$

- If the process average and the target are the same value, C_{pm} will be the Same as Cpk. If the average drifts from the target value, C_{pm} will be less than the Cpk value.

Calculations of process capability are based on the assumption that the data are taken from a normal distribution. Doers should be aware of the relationship of the two most commonly used measures, Cp and Cpk, which are considered to be measures of long-term capability. Together, these two measures provide information regarding the process variation and where the process is centered in relation to the specification limits. If the values are the same, the process is centered. The process is less centered as the difference between these two values increases. The less centered the process, the lower the Cpk will be and the greater the probability of measures outside the specification limits.

15.4 Qualitative and Quantitative Analysis

Quantitative data means either that measurements were taken or that a count was made, such as counting the number of defective pieces removed (inspected out), the number of customer complaints, or the number of cycles of a molding press observed during a time period. In short, the data are expressed as a measurement or an amount.

In contrast, qualitative data refers to the nature, kind, or attribute of an observation Qualitative data must be unbiased and traceable. Quantitative information help in a direct comparison between the information and the requirements.

A. Patterns and Trends:

- **Pattern analysis** involves the collection of data in a way that readily reveals any kind of clustering that may occur.
- No specific single tool exists to determine patterns and trends. Patterns and trends can used to help determine whether a problem is a systemic issue or not.

- **Line/Trend graphs** connect points that represent pairs of numeric data, to show how one variable of the pair is a function of the other. As a matter of convention, independent variables are plotted on the horizontal axis, and dependent variables are plotted on the vertical axis. *Line graphs are used to show changes in data over time.*
- A trend is indicated when a series of points heads up or down. Nonrandom patterns indicate a trend or tendency.
- **Bar graphs** also portray the relationship or comparison between pairs of variables, but one of the variables need not be numeric. Each bar in a bar graph represents a separate or discrete, value. Bar graphs can be used to identify differences between sets of data.
- **Pie charts** are used to depict proportions of data or information in order to understand how they make up the whole. The entire circle, or "pie," represents 100 percent of the data. The circle is divided into "slices," with each segment being proportional to the numeric quantity in each class or category.
- **Matrices are two-dimensional tables** showing the relationship between two sets of information. They can be used to show the logical connecting points between performance criteria and implementing actions, or between required actions and personnel responsible for those actions. In this way, matrices are used for determining what actions and/or personnel have the greatest impact on an organization's mission.

15.5 Measures of Statistical Tools Analysis

When you use the correct statistical tools at the right time, your manufacturing processes become more understandable, they achieve a higher quality level, and you become better prepared to explain how your processes work to others. For regulatory inspections, you'll be well-prepared to demonstrate the correct use of statistical quality tools in your response. More important, ensuring that your processes are producing the quality your customers need means that you won't receive a warning letter in the first place.

CHAPTER 16

Application of Different Quality Tools in Investigation of Non-Conformance Observations

Introduction

The pharmaceutical environment today is changing quickly due to globalization, increased competition, cost constraints, demands for efficiency, and development of international regulation, supply chain complexity, and product/process complexity. Quality tools describes a systematic, efficient, and effective way of ensuring that manufacturing systems and equipment are fit for intended use , and that risk to product quality, and consequently to patient safety , are effectively managed to the extent that these are affected by systems and equipment.

***Types of Non-Conformance Events*:** A non-conformance means that something went wrong - a problem has occurred and needs to be addressed with corrective and preventive actions. Documented procedure control should be available for the handling of non-conformance with to define controls, responsibility and authority. When the nonconforming is corrected it must be re-verified to demonstrate conformity.

Sufficient trained personnel and resources should be made available for the handling, assessment, investigation and review of complaints and quality defects and for implementing any risk-reducing actions.

16.1 Deviation Management

Deviation Management is a part of QMS providing efficient support for controlling deviation incidents, implementing corrective measures, helping avoid their recurrence, and for taking a proactive approach to continuous quality improvement.

"Any departure from the approved process or procedure is called deviation" Type of deviations are :

- ***Planned Deviations*:** Planned and know before its occurs.
- ***Unplanned Deviations*:** Occur without intimation.

A. Steps Involved in Deviation Investigation:

- Login of Deviations and description.
- Event Detection and investigation.
- Risk Analysis and Impact Assessment.
- Deviation Categorization.
- Root cause analysis.
- CAPA.
- Efficacy of corrective action and conclusion.
- Verification and closure.

Deviation Management is a part of QMS providing efficient support for controlling deviation incidents, implementing corrective measures, helping avoid their recurrence, and for taking a proactive approach to continuous quality improvement.

B. Deviation Categorization:

- ***Major Deviations*:** When the deviation affects a quality attribute, a critical process parameter, an equipment or instrument critical for process or control, of which the impact to patients (or personnel/environment) is unlikely, the deviation is categorized as Major requiring immediate action, investigation, and documented.
- ***Critical Deviations*:** When the deviation affects a quality attribute, a critical process parameter, an equipment or instrument critical for process or control, of which the impact to patients (or personnel or environment) is highly probable, including life threatening situation, the deviation is categorized as Critical requiring immediate action, investigated, and documented.
- ***Minor Deviation*:** When the deviation does not affect any quality attribute, a critical process parameter, or an equipment or instrument critical for process or control, it

would be categorized as Minor **Quality** Risk Management can be used for the identification of product attributes and operational parameters which are critical to manufacturing operations in order to identify in advance their associated risks.

16.2 Complaint

Complaint means any written, electronic, or oral communication that alleges deficiencies related to the identity, quality, durability, reliability, safety, effectiveness, or performance of a device after it is released for distribution.

All quality related complaints, whether received orally or in writing, must be recorded and investigated according to a written procedure.

Complaint records should include:

- Name and address of complainant.
- Name (and, where appropriate, title) and phone number of person submitting the complaint.
- Complaint nature (including name and batch number of the API).
- Date complaint is received.
- Action initially taken (including dates and identity of person taking the action).
- Any follow-up action taken.
- Response provided to the originator of complaint (including date response sent); and
- Final decision on intermediate or API batch or lot.
- Records of complaints should be retained in order to evaluate trends, product-related frequencies, and severity with a view to taking additional, and if appropriate, immediate corrective action.

A. Steps Involved in Complaint Handling:

- Login of Complaint and description.
- Investigation of Complaint by cross function team: Document review, Previous history, similar type of complaint, trend analysis, Laboratory analysis, reserve sample checks, Production and Packing records review, Counterfeit product.

- Root cause analysis.
- Risk Analysis and Impact Assessment.
- CAPA.
- Conclusion.
- Feed back to customer or complainant.
- Efficacy of corrective action and conclusion.
- Verification and closure.

16.3 Recall

Recall means a firm's removal or correction of a marketed product. Aprroved procedure should be available. Recalled products should be identified and stored separately in a secure area. The progress of the recall process should be recorded until closure and a final report issued, including a reconciliation between the delivered and recovered quantities of the concerned products/batches.

A. Classification of Recall:

Recalls are classified based on health hazard.

- Class I - a situation in which there is a reasonable probability that the use of, or exposure to, a violative product will cause serious adverse health consequences or death.
- Class II - a situation in which use of, or exposure to, a violative product may cause temporary or medically reversible adverse health consequences or where the probability of serious adverse health consequences is remote.
- Class III - a situation in which use of, or exposure to, a violative product is not likely to cause adverse health consequences.

B. Recall Strategy:

Recall strategy means a planned course of action to be taken in conducting a specific recall, which addresses the depth of recall, need for public warnings, and extent of effectiveness checks for the recall. Depth of recall (Consumer or user level, Retailer) depends on results of health hazard evaluation. Following information should be available for recall marketed product.

- Identity of the product involved, batch number/lot number.
- Reason for the removal or correction and the date and circumstances under which the product deficiency or possible deficiency was discovered.
- Evaluation of the risk associated with the deficiency or possible deficiency.
- Total amount of such products produced and/or the time span of the production.
- Total amount of such products estimated to be in distribution channels.
- Distribution information, including the number of direct accounts and, where necessary, the identity of the direct accounts.
- A copy of the firm's recall communication if any has issued, or a proposed communication if none has issued.
- Proposed strategy for conducting the recall.
- Name and telephone number of the firm official who should be contacted concerning the recall.
- A recall communication can be accomplished by telegrams, mailgrams, or first class letters conspicuously marked, preferably in bold red type, on the letter and the envelope: "medical device recall [or correction]". The letter and the envelope should be also marked: "urgent" for class I and class II recalls and, when appropriate, for class III recalls. Telephone calls or other personal contacts should ordinarily be confirmed by one of the above methods and/or documented in an appropriate manner.

C. **Recall Communication:**

A recall communication should be written in accordance with the following information.

- Be brief and to the point;
- Identify clearly the product, size, lot number(s), code(s) or serial number(s) and any other pertinent descriptive information to enable accurate and immediate identification of the product;
- Explain concisely the reason for the recall and the hazard involved, if any;

- Provide specific instructions on what should be done with respect to the recalled products; and
- Provide a ready means for the recipient to report to the recalling firm whether it has any of the product, e.g., by sending a postage-paid, self-addressed postcard or by allowing the recipient to place a collect call to the recalling firm.

D. Recall Status Reports:

The recall status report should contain the following information:

- Number of consignees notified of the recall, and date and method of notification.
- Number of consignees responding to the recall communication and quantity of products on hand at the time it was received.
- Number of consignees that did not.
- Number of products returned or corrected by each consignee contacted and the quantity of products accounted for.
- Number and results of effectiveness checks that were made.
- Estimated time frames for completion of the recall.

E. Effectiveness Checks:

The effectiveness checks is to verify that all consignees have received notification about the recall and have taken appropriate action. Consignees may be contacted by personal visits, telephone calls, letters, or a combination thereof. A guide entitled "Methods for Conducting Recall Effectiveness Checks" that describes the use of these different methods is available from FDA. The recalling firm will ordinarily be responsible for conducting effectiveness checks, but FDA will assist in this task where necessary and appropriate. The recall strategy will specify the method(s) to be used for and the level of effectiveness checks that will be conducted, as follows:

- Level A--100 percent of the total number of consignees to be contacted;
- Level B--Some percentage of the total number of consignees to be contacted, which percentage is to be determined on a

case-by-case basis, but is greater that 10 percent and less than 100 percent of the total number of consignees;

- Level C--10 percent of the total number of consignees to be contacted;
- Level D--2 percent of the total number of consignees to be contacted; or
- Level E--No effectiveness checks

The effectiveness of the arrangements in place for recalls should be periodically evaluated to confirm that they remain robust and fit for use. Such evaluations should extend to both within office-hour situations as well as out-of-office hour situations and, when performing such evaluations, consideration should be given as to whether mock-recall actions should be performed. This evaluation should be documented and justified.

16.4 Out of Specification (OOS)

The term OOS results include all test results that fall out of the specifications or acceptance criteria established in item or product. OOS must be thorough, timely, unbiased, well documented and scientifically sound. OOS investigation consist of two phase:

- Phase I : Laboratory investigation.
- Phase II : Full-Scale OOS investigation.

A. Phase l: Laboratory Investigation:

In Phase 1 Analyst report the OOS to laboratory supervisor .Supervisor log OOS. Initial investigation is carried out by involving analyst by interviewing him / her for correct procedure, data, calculation chemicals, standards, glassware used. Checklist can be prepared for the same. This phase also includes verification by reinjection the initial preparation for hypotheses regarding what might have happen such as dilution error , instrument error. Original sample must not be destroy till the investigation is completed, if the test solution stability is less , then justification for same must be documented with back up data.

- If clear laboratory error is identified, the firm must determine the source of that error and take corrective and preventive action. All the laboratory assessment must be documented. Initial investigation must be completed in defined time with scientifically sound conclusion. After conclusion In-valid the previous data.

- If clear laboratory error is not identified or un-clear a full-scale investigation must be carried out .Both the initial laboratory assessment and following OOS investigation must be documented fully. In this case initial data must not be done in- valid.

B. Phase II: Full Scale Investigation:

- When the initial assessment does not determine the laboratory error caused the OOS result and testing results appear to be accurate, a full –scale investigation using predefined procedure must be conducted. This investigation may consist of a production review and/or laboratory work. The objective of such an investigation must be to identify the root cause analysis of the OOS result and take appropriate corrective and preventive action. A full-scale investigation must include a review of production and sampling procedures, and will often include additional laboratory testing..Such investigation must be give high priority.
- A full-scale OOS investigation must consist of a timely, through and well documented review. A written record of the review must include.

  a. ***Production Review***: The investigation must be conducted by Quality assurance along with other department including manufacturing, process developments maintenance and engineering. Potential problem must be identified and investigated. The records and documentation of the manufacturing process must be fully reviewed to determine the possible cause of the OOS result.

     - A clear statement of the reason for the investigation.
     - A summary of the aspects of the manufacturing process that may have caused the problem.
     - The results of documentation review, with the assignment of actual or probable cause.
     - The results of a review made to determine if the problem has occurred previously.

- A description action taken.
- If this part of the OOS investigation confirms the OOS results and is successful in identifying the root cause, the OOS investigation may be terminated and the product rejected. However a failure investigation must be completed with predefined time. If any material is reprocessed after additional testing, the investigation must include comments and the signatures of appropriate production and quality control and quality assurance personnel.

b. ***Additional Laboratory Testing*: A** full-scale OOS investigation may include additional laboratory testing. A number of practices are used during the laboratory phase of an investigation. These include retesting a portion of the original sample and re-sampling.

- ***Retesting*:** The sample used for retesting must be taken from same homogeneous material that originally collected from the lot, tested and yielded the OOS results .For a liquid, it may be from the original unit liquid product or composite of the liquid product and for solid, it may be from the same sample composite prepared for the original sample.
- ***Decision*** of retest must be based on the objectives of testing and scientific judgment. It is often important for the predefined retesting plan to include retests performed by an analyst other than the one who performed the original test. A second analyst performing a retest must be at least as experienced and qualified in the method as the original analyst. The maximum number of retests to be performed on sample must be specified in advance in a written standard operating procedure. The number of retest must not be adjusted depending on the results obtained.
- If **no** laboratory or calculation errors are identified in the first test, there is no scientific basis for invalidating initial OOS results in favor of passing results. All test results, both passing and suspect

must be reported and considered in batch release decisions.

- *Resampling*: After Quality Assurance approval for resamples the original sample from an batch where OOS is occurred. Resampling must be performed by the same qualified, validated methods that are used for the initial sample. However, if the investigation determines that initial sampling methods was inherently inadequate; a nee accurate sampling method must be developed, documented, and reviewed and approved by the quality assurance.
- *Reporting Testing Results*: Averaging the results of the original test that prompted during an OOS investigation and additional retest or results obtained during the OOS investigation is not appropriate because it hides variability among the individual sample.
- *Conclusion the Investigation*: To conclude the investigation, the results must be investigated and the findings of the investigation, including retest results, must be interpreted to evaluate the batch and reach a decision regarding release or rejection. A confirmed OOS result indicates that the batch does not meet established standards or specification must be rejected and disposed with proper documentation. Impact on the other batches and product must be studied.

  For inconclusive investigations-in case where an investigation I(1) does not reveal a cause for the OOS test results and (2) does not confirm the OOS results must be give full consideration in batch or lot disposal decision.

16.5 Field Alter Report (FAR)

Field Alter report is submitted to USFDA regulation within 3 working days for those product that are subjected of approved full abbreviated new drug applications, which are not meeting approved specification. OOS test results on these products are considered to be one kind of "information concerns any failure".

Unless the OOS results on the distributed batch is found to be invalid within 3 days, an initial FAR must be submitted follow up FAR must be submitted when the OOS investigation is completed.

16.6 Out of Trend (OOT)

An out of trend result is the result that does not follow the expected trend, either in comparison with other batches or with respect to previous results collected.

Trend limits is to be generated on sufficient analytical data by averaging the value. Variable values must not be average as average value may hide variability and may result into in appropriate limits. The greater trend limits must not be exceeding the release limits. The limit can be by finalized on complied date from all the batches by approaches such as 3 sigma or 5 sigma or 6 sigma. The back update must be attached for trend analysis. Trend must be reviewed periodically. OOT investigation can be performed as per OOS investigation.

16.7 Investigations Tools

Different investigation tools can be used for the investigation of non-conformance and to have effective CAPA.

A. Root Cause Analysis (RCA):

Root Cause Investigation is a powerful tool used for quality improvement. Among the different tools available for Root Cause Investigation, the "5 Whys" and "Ishikawa Fish Bone Diagram" are the simplest and most used ones. The "5 Whys" refers to a series of sequential questions (i.e. each response given is asked "why", normally from 3 up to 5 times). This exercise allows a thorough understanding of the underlying or root causes of the deviation, which may be related to a systemic problem.

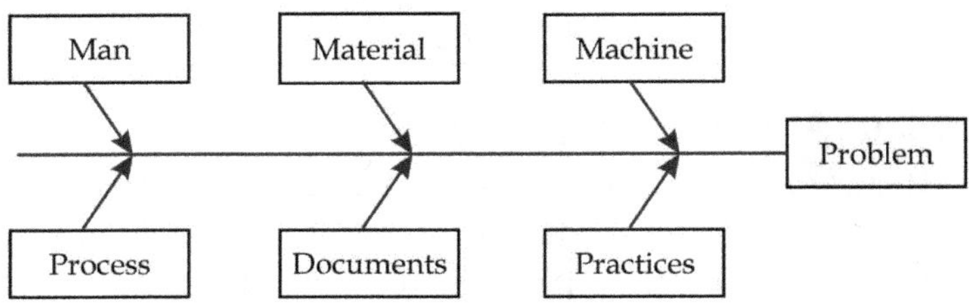

Figure 16.1 Fish bone diagram.

The Fish bone diagram is a cause-effect type of analysis where the product / process is the main spine, the effect is the actual non- conformance, and the secondary spines are the different factors or causes that could have affected or "caused" (i.e., materials, controls, personnel, equipment, procedures, etc.).

B. Corrective and Preventive Action (CAPA):

The root cause investigation process is a key step in handling nonconformance and provide objective evidence to implement corrective and possibly preventive actions as part of the CAPA system. CAPA is concept that focuses on investigating and correcting discrepancies and attempting to prevent recurrence. CAPA has three concepts.

a. ***Remedial action***: Root cause analysis with corrective and preventive action to prevent recurrence

b. ***Preventive action***: to prevent initial occurrence.

c. ***Corrective action***: A corrective action is a term that encompasses the process of reacting to product problems, customer complaints or other nonconformities and fixing them. The process includes;

- Reviewing and defining the problem or nonconformance,
- Finding the cause of the problem,
- Developing an action plan to correct the problem,
- Developing an action plan to correct the problem and prevent recurrence,
- Implementing an action plan to correct the problem and prevent a recurrence,
- Implementing the plan,
- Evaluating the effectiveness of the correction.

d. ***Preventive actions***: A preventive action is process for detecting potential problems or nonconformance's and eliminating them. The process includes

- Identify the potential problem or non -conformance,
- Find the cause of the potential problem
- Develop a plan to prevent the occurrence
- Implement the plan
- Review the actions taken and effectiveness is preventing the problem.

e. **Steps Involved in CAPA Procedure:**

- The identification of the problem, non conformity or the problem, nonconformity or incident.
- An Evaluation of the magnitude of the problem and potential impact on the company ,
- The development of an investigation procedures with assignments of responsibility,
- Performing a thorough Analysis of the problem with appropriate documentation
- Creating an Action Plan listing all the tasks that must be completed to correct and /or prevent the problem.
- Implementation the plan.
- A thorough Follow up with verification of the completion of all tasks and assessment of the appropriateness and effectiveness of the actions taken.
- Close of CAPA after effectiveness of the action taken.

C. **Risk Management Program:**

Risk is defined as the combination of the probability of occurrence of harm and the severity of that harm, and could be followed by the probability of detection. A risk-based quality management system consists of the identification of hazards and the analysis and evaluation of risks associated with exposure to those hazards through a multidisciplinary approach. QRM consists of three main steps which actually work as a continuous improvement cycle:

- Identification of Hazards, based on well-defined process description, and adequate sources of information (e.g. historical data; description of the possible consequences). It addresses the question "What might go wrong?".
- Risk Analysis estimates the risk associated with the identified hazard/s. "It is the qualitative or quantitative process of linking the likelihood (probability) of occurrence and severity of harms; in some risk management tools, the ability to detect the harm (i.e. detectability) also factors in the estimation of risk".

- Risk Evaluation "compares the identified and analyzed risk against given risk criteria and the strength of evidence for all three of the fundamental questions".
- Risk Review the effectiveness of the risk management process should be reviewed periodically based on meaningful information.
- Risk Communication sharing of the outcome of the deployment of QRM

a. **Quality Risk Management Tools:**

Quality risk management is a process that supports science-based and practical decisions when integrated into quality systems. Different tolls are used for effective quality risk management which can facilitate better and more informed decisions. Following are some quality risk management tools ,but not limited to;

- Basic risk management facilitation methods: Some of the simple techniques that are commonly used to structure risk management by organizing data and facilitating decision-making are: Flowcharts; Check Sheets; Process Mapping; Cause and Effect Diagrams (also called an Ishikawa diagram or fish bone diagram).
- Failure Mode Effects Analysis (FMEA);
- Failure Mode, Effects and Criticality Analysis (FMECA);
- Fault Tree Analysis (FTA);
- Hazard Analysis and Critical Control Points (HACCP);
- Hazard Operability Analysis (HAZOP);
- Preliminary Hazard Analysis (PHA);
- Risk ranking and filtering;
- Supporting statistical tools.

There are several QRM tools from which Failure Modes Effects Analysis (FMEA) is commonly applied due to its versatility. This tool is used for identifying potential failures and to examine the impact of deviations on product quality, and to propose more adequate corrective and preventive actions. The QRM is ideally performed prospectively.

FMEA includes the following aspects:

- **Probability,** or frequency of occurrence.
- **Detectability,** includes methods to detect deviations or their associated parameters
- **Severity**or how significant the deviation is in terms of impact of the deviation on product quality and patient´s safety.

The output of a risk assessment may be a combination of quantitative and qualitative estimation of risk. As part of FMEA, a risk score or "Risk Prioritization Number or RPN". RPN is calculated by multiplying Probability (P), Detectability (D) and Severity (S), which are individually categorized and scored as described below in Table 16.1.

Table 16.1 Risk assessment scoring table.

Risk	P*- Probability		D*-Detectability		S*-Severity	
Extremely low	2	Highly improbable to occur				
Low	4	Improbable to occur	6	Control system in place has a low probability of detecting the defect or its effects	2	Minor GMP non-compliance; no possible impact on Patient, yield or on production capability.
Moderate	6	Probable to occur	4	Control system in place could detect the defect or its effects	4	Significant GMP non-compliance; possible impact on patient; moderate impact on yield or production capability.
High	8	Highly probable to occur	2	Control system in place has a high probability of detecting the defect or its effects	6	Major GMP non-compliance; probable impact on patient; high impact on yield or production capability.
Non existent			8	There is no control system to detect the defect		

Table 16.1 *Contd..*

Risk	P*- Probability		D*-Detectability		S*-Severity	
Critical					54	Serious GMP non-compliance; Probable serious harm or death; critical impact on yield or production capability.
(*) The scoring should be assigned in an objective well justified manner as applicable by the FMEA team, which should be carefully selected based on scientific background, product knowledge and experience						

Possible interpretation of the RPN used to categorize:

- ***Critical***: RPN between 216 (6 x 6 x 6) and 512 (8 x 8 x 8) is considered a critical risk and must be addressed immediately and treated as a critical.
- ***Major***: RPN between 64 and 216 is considered major risk and must be addressed in a timely manner as a major.
- ***Minor***: RPN between 8 and 64 indicates a low risk and must be addressed in a timely manner as a minor deviation.

16.8 Verification Program

A **systematic** approach must be defined to verify that manufacturing systems, acting singly or in combination, are fit for intended use, have been properly installed and are operating correctly. This verification approach must be defined and documented. The extent of verification and level of detail of documentation must be based on risk, including those associated with product quality and patient safety, and the complexity and novelty of manufacturing system.

CHAPTER 17

New Approach to the Internal Audit from Traditional to Risk based Approach

Introduction

The complexity of today's pharmaceutical market requires more efficient drug development and production throughout the product Lifecycle along with Data management to meets the quality requirements. IA is an important performance indicator used to identify the gaps and correct them on timely basis to meets the quality requirements. IA should formally design to identify and manage the risks to drive realistic continual improvement.

ISO 9001 refers to a "Plan-Do-Check-Act" methodology for addressing processes in a quality management system. This methodology can be applied two ways in regards to IAs. The audit itself may be considered a process in which one plans by developing an auditing procedure and audit schedule, does the audit, checks that the audit process worked properly, and then acts upon any observations of the audit process. Secondly, the auditing process can also be used as a part of the checking step in the Plan-Do-Check-Act methodology. The Act step is the corrective and preventive actions taken as part of a continuous improvement of the audited process. Audits should not be viewed negatively as a means of finding weaknesses or problems, but in a positive light by looking an opportunity for continuous improvement in operations. Of course audit results are only one piece of the total picture that management should consider when performing management reviews of operations, but they should serve as unbiased observations of opportunities for improvement.

17.1 Traditional Approach to IA

Traditional IA was a singular functional and location view that fed a static audit plan.

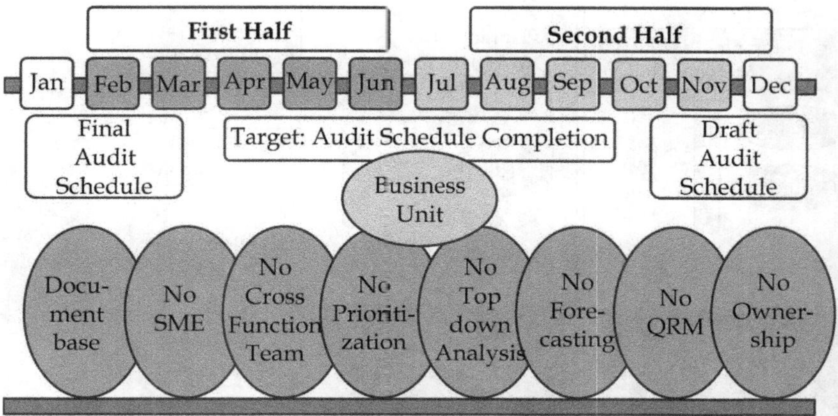

Figure 17.1 Historical Annual Process Map.

Traditionally IA were conducted as on periodic basis and percentage of audit recommendation was implemented by management was 0-40%. Auditing staff for IA was also responsible for day to day activity in the organization. So IA was given as second priority of work (Figure 1: Historical Annual Process Map).

17.2 Forecasting Approach to IA

In 21st Century IA Principles & Techniques shall be depends on Preventative, Detective, Corrective, Directive and Compensating with IA methods such as Organizational Controls, Operational Controls, Personnel Controls, Periodic Review Controls, and Facilities & Equipment Controls. Risk assessment tool will help the organization in continuous improvement, increased enterprise wide influence, End to end involvement in risk decisions, direct access to board or risk committees, Identification and mitigation of emerging risks.

Risk assessment compliance with help to meet regulatory expectation.

IA is a unique activity which involves a combination of audit approaches and techniques. These include interviews, document reviews, sampling, testing of controls, and analysis of transaction, processes and management information. The IA strategy play important role during IA activity such as planning, examination, evaluation and effectiveness of the system, audit conclusion, review, communication and follow-up.

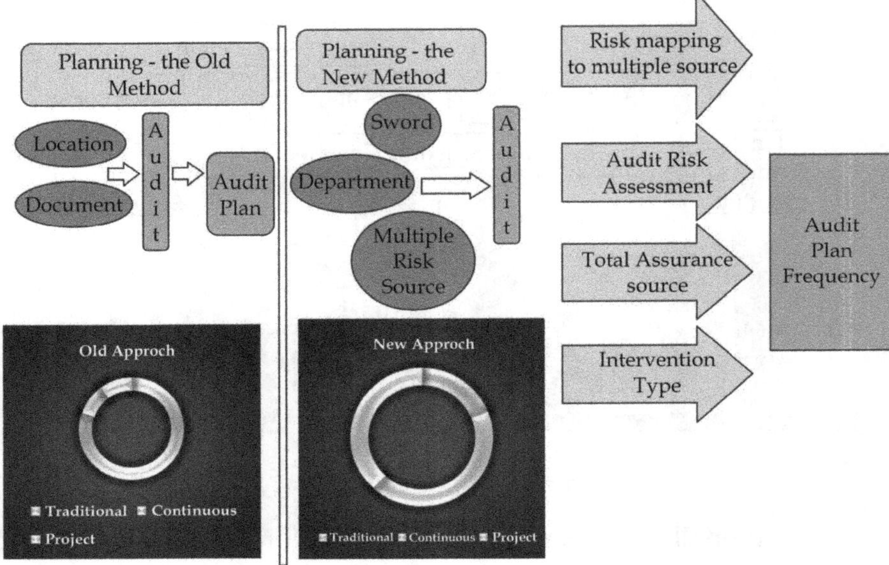

Figure 17.2 Forecasting Approach to IA Map: Old to New Quality Approach.

17.3 Benefits of QRM to IA Program

- Proactive management and Transparency of information
- Management override, Governance Risk control and Harmonies change management.
- Effectiveness and efficiency of operations and programs.
- Compliance with laws, regulations, policies, procedures and contracts.
- Facilitate risk-based regulatory oversight and optimization of resources for assessment and inspection.
- Emphasize use of the control strategy as a key component of the regulatory commitment.
- Help assure supply reliability by enabling strategic management.
- Keeps the team focused on continuously considering and assessing risk.

17.4 IA Approach to Organization

1. Quality System
2. Facilities and Equipment System
3. Production System
4. Materials System
5. Lab Control System
6. Packaging and Labeling System

Figure 17.3 The Quality Six Systems Model.

IA shall be conducted by different types of tools such as usage of flowchart, questionnaires, risk control matrixes, policy, procedural manual, vertical audit, horizontal audit, sampling based or system based. Approach of IA shall depends on the risk, loop falls and types of non-conformance (11). System based or risk base approach can be selected for IA as mostly useful tool to identify the gap in the organization.

I. System based Approach:

The systems based IA program have the ability to assess whether each of the systems is in a state of control. The quality system audits consist of individual inspection of Quality System, Facilities and Equipment System, Materials System, Production System, Packaging and Labeling System, Laboratory System to correct the non-conformity. (Refer Figure 2: The Quality system module). System base IA can also be performed on fragile system identified during past audit. System review is a key component in any healthy quality system to ensure its continuing suitability, adequacy, and effectiveness. Under a quality system, senior managers are expected to conduct reviews of the whole quality system according to a planned schedule. Such a review typically includes both an assessment of the product as well as customer needs.

The review should consider at least the following:

- The appropriateness of the quality policy and its objectives.
- The results of audits and other assessments.
- Customer feedback, including complaints.
- The analysis of data trending results.
- The status of actions to prevent potential problems or their recurrence.
- Any follow-up actions from previous management reviews.
- Any changes in business practices or environment that may affect the quality system.

- Whether product characteristics meet the customer's needs.
- Science-based approaches.

System based audit during IA can be approach as;

A. Full Inspection Option: Quality System + NLT 3 other systems
- Initial establishment inspection
- Previous inspection findings, non compliances
- Significant changes since last inspection (New technologies, equipment's, facilities.
- Follow up to non-conformities.
- Revert to an abbreviated option with district concurrence.

B. Abbreviated Inspection Option: Quality System + NMT 2 other systems
- Good history.
- No major changes to operations.
- No pattern of recalls and problems.
- When not using the full inspection option.
- Surveillance inspections.
- Adequate for routine coverage.
- Rotate system with the Abbreviated option-District will monitor.

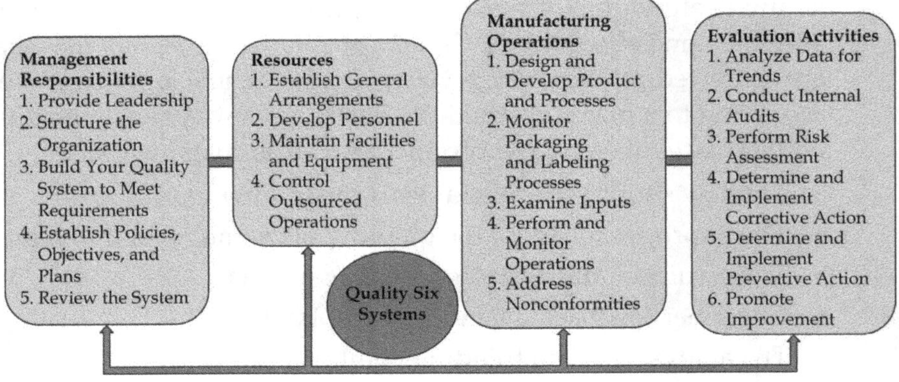

Figure 17.4 Linked bases approach.

II. Linked based - Process Approach:

Linked **based** internal audit approach depends on six-system inspection model includes how the cGMP and the concepts of modern quality systems are linked. The new six-system inspection model shows the quality system and the five manufacturing systems. Under the Quality Systems Model, the Agency recommends that senior managers ensure that the quality system they design and implement provides clear organizational guidance and facilitates the systematic evaluation of issues. Refer Figure 4: Linked bases Approach.

III. Risk based Approach for IA Program:

New era for self-inspection by implementation of QRM .The concept of risk management is a major focus of the "Pharmaceutical cGMPs for the 21st Century" initiative. Risk management can guide the setting of specifications and process parameters. Risk assessment is also used in determining the need for discrepancy investigations and corrective actions and how to prioritize them. Adoption of risk assessment approach will promote innovation and continual improvement, and strengthen quality assurance and reliable supply of product. Risk-based approach can apply for assessing changes across the life cycle, identification of several gaps. IA with Quality risk management and knowledge management achieve product realization, maintain a state of control, and facilitate continual improvement. The purpose of risk based approach to IA program can be applied in two-fold as:

- To design IA as a quality risk management tool that can provide the objective evidence to the management about whether or not the current and potential risks to quality are effectively managed to acceptable levels. Management then can judge the effectiveness of process and functions within the quality system.
- Efficient inspection workload and resource management focusing on those areas within the quality system that present higher risk to the quality of medicinal product with aim of meeting the quality objective.

IV. Forensic Audit:

Forensic audit is a process of investigation where or not fraud is happen against approved standards. Forensic Audits covers a broad spectrum of activities of organization. Main objective of forensic audit is to find out whether all system, process, data governance system meets the regulatory/ procedure/ policy/ standards requirements.

Forensic audit shall be conducted to know data integrity in current good manufacturing practice (cGMP) for drugs. Forensic audit is conducted to verify the completeness, consistency, and accuracy of data .Complete, consistent, and accurate data should be attributable, legible, contemporaneously recorded, original or a true copy, and accurate (ALCOA) .Forensic audit can be conducted on static documents (fixed-data document such as a paper record or an electronic image), and dynamic record (format allows interaction between the user and the record content).

Forensic audit many be conducted in ways, similar to the process of conducting a normal audit, but with some additional considerations shall be taken such as;

- Identifying the type of fraud that has been operating.
- How long it has been operating for,
- How the fraud was concealed for the duration,
- Identifying the fraudster(s) involved,
- Quantifying and gathering evidence.

Forensic audit can be done is two ways Reactive Forensic Audit and Proactive Forensic Audit.

- **Reactive Forensic Auditing:** To investigate suspected fraud so as to prove the suspicions, and suspicions are proves by findings by evidence and present evidence in an acceptable format.
- **Proactive Forensic Auditing:** Forensic auditing in this sense could be viewed from different aspects depending on its application such as regulatory compliance.

V. For-Cause-Audit:

For-Cause-Audit is an audit conducted anything other than a routine internal audit. For cause audit is to investigate a specific problem such as Field Alert report, recall adverse events or other events. For-Cause-Audit is an in-depth examination of all components including but not limited to records, documents, interview etc.

Any above tools can be selected for internal audit to know the loop falls and take corrective and preventive action.

17.5 Planning

Risk management can be applied for IA planning ·The application of the risk management allows the estimation of the risk associated with areas within quality system and determine the scope, frequency, time, number of inspectors and allocation of inspectors to particular area based on SME, which help in risk-based inspection planning and better utilization of man power. During the risk assessment to IA schedule risk assessment process shall be done such as Figure 17.5.

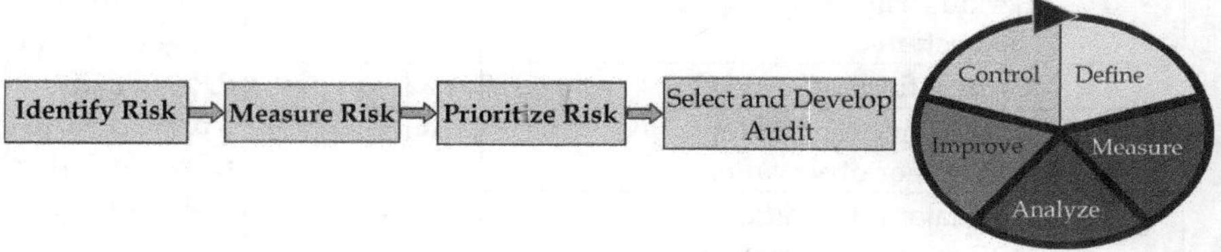

Figure 17.5 Quality risk assessment.

Quality risk Assessment. Planning of the IA shall be based on the prioritization and risk assed .Three primary methods can be selected for the annual audit plan.

- Cycle approach
- Risk based approach
- Cycle-Based Risk approach

Risk can be identified based on quality risk matrix such as the historical data of IAs, regulatory observation, and regulation guideline updating, warning letters or other factors as;

- Complexity of the site, manufacturing process, Batch Failure rate, Process Capability/Performance,
- Critical areas,
- Major changes in facility, equipment & process,
- Compliance status and history of unit,
- Complaints and Recalls received,
- the inherent risk of the drug manufactured,
- The inspection frequency and history of the establishment,
- Laboratory failure investigation rate/Invalidated Out-of-Specification (OOS) Rate,
- CAPA Effectiveness,
- Warning letters.

Simple approach could be assigning a numerical descriptive value of1 (low), 2(moderate) and 3(high) to established categories for the selection risk factors. The estimated values for risk factors could also be multiplied by significance-weighting factors to give a total. (Table 17.1- Approach to risk rating)

Table 17.1 Risk rating level

Risk Rating level	Input from current inspection findings	Internal frequency	Approach
0	Serious triggering outside the inspection cycle	Immediate	• Number of regulatory audits • Results of previous IAs • Fragile system identified
1	Critical finding	Twice in year	
2	> 6 major observation > 10 minor observation	Twice in year	
3	< 6 major observation < 10 minor observation	Yearly	
4	No Critical or Major finding or < 10 minor observation	Yearly	
5	No Critical or Major finding from current or previous inspection and < 6 other finding each.	Yearly	

Use of quality metrics will support to understanding of the inherent risk of manufacturing establishments and products. The collection of these data will help to direct our inspections. These metrics may provide a basis for IA to use improved risk based principles to determine the appropriate audit scheduling. Once all risk have been mapped to relevant audits, the audits are then ranked from highest to lowest base on audit score. The annual plan shall be chosen based on the percentage of "total risk". Understanding the top compliance risk is an important parameter in risk assessment audit scheduling. The compliance risk assessment will help the organization under standard the full range of its risks exposure, including likelihood that a risk event occur, the reason it may occur, and the potential severity of its impact. The risk associated can estimate by using different tools. Use of available tools is to understand processes, improve processes / products.

17.6 Audit Sampling

Audit sampling plays important role to collect evidences to support observation and opinions. The type of sampling used and number of items selected should be based on the auditors understanding of the relative risk and exposures of the areas audited. Sampling involves some selection of certain sections of the data or population based on its quantitative or qualitative factors. Thus, the IA team must undertake statistically backed sample selection technique to ensure designing efficient samples, measuring sufficient evidence and evaluating results with objectivity.

Allowable Risk is calculated as: AR = IR × CR × DR

- AR = the allowable audit risk that a material misstatement might remain undetected
- IR = Inherent risk, the risk of a material misstatement in an assertion, assuming there were no related controls.
- CR = Control risk, the risk that a material misstatement that could occur in an assertion will not be prevented or detected on a timely basis by internal control.
- DR = Detection risk, the risk that the auditors' procedures will fail to detect a material misstatement if it exists.

  The sample size selected affects the level of sampling risk of the sample. Every increase in sample size reduces the sampling risk and allowance for sampling risk. The sample size is generally directly proportionate to the characteristics of the population and an increase in the population leads to an increase in the sample size. The different methodologies available for statistically based selection of sample size such as Random Sampling, Consecutive Sampling (snapshot: first or last), Consecutive Sampling (Systematic sampling), Haphazard Sampling (The Haphazard Sampling method means selecting items on an arbitrary basis, but without any), Block Sampling (Time period) and Stratification sampling (dividing the population homogenously).

17.7 Audit Tools

Horizontal or vertical IA can be conducted to check the organization state of control. Vertical audits covers activities within given function or physical area, whereas, horizontal audit address a single contract, project or product Techniques such as interviewing, examine the records, observation, drawback and Pitfall can be used.

17.8 Audit Evidence and Analysis Phase

During IA sufficient, relevant, reliable and useful information shall be collected· Different types of evidence can be obtained during the course of IA such as physical, testimonial, documentary or analytical evidence to support audit observation. Sampling tools such as statically or probability, Attribute, Variable and judgment can be used during IA. For audit analysis root cause model for IA can be used. (Figure 17.4: Root cause Model for IA).

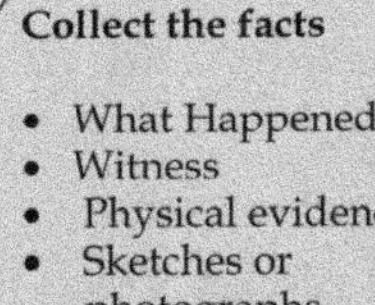

Figure 17.6 Root cause model for IA.

17.9 Audit CLOSE-OUT and FOLLOW-UP

At the conclusion of the audit, there should be a close-out meeting to discuss the observations. Ensure that all parties have a clear understanding of the observations and any commitments to corrective actions. Timeframe should be provided for when the audit report will be made available and when responses to observations will be provided. Schedules for completing corrective actions should be developed. Depending on the observations made and the commitments to corrective actions, a follow-up audit may be necessary. If a decision is made to not conduct a follow-up audit, the corrective actions should be reviewed in any future audits. Documentation of the rationale for not conducting a follow-up audit can be useful for future audits; unless the audit procedure clearly defines when follow-up audits are or are not required. Preventive as well as corrective actions should be taken to address unfavorable observations. Preventive actions are focused on improving the quality system so that the same unfavorable observations are not repeated.

CHAPTER 18

Quality by Design (QbD) Approach in the Product Life Cycle

Introduction

QbD is comprehensive understanding of the product and manufacturing process to consistently deliver the intended performance of the product throughout its life cycle.

"The pharmaceutical Quality by Design (QbD) is a systematic approach to development that begins with predefined objectives and emphasizes product and process understanding and process control, based on sound science and quality risk management."

Principle of QbD Concepts is Zero defects and is based on the:

- Systematic approach to develop product on realisation by multivariate experiment.
- Manufacturing process adjustable within the design space.
- Establish and maintain a state of control.
- Focus on control strategy and robustness of the process to facilitate continual improvement.
- Knowledge management and quality risk management based decisions.
- Product ownership.
- Continuous Improvement Cycle based on "PDCA Cycle": PLAN (Plan the steps), DO (Perform the steps), CHECK (Analyse the results) and ACT (Use the results).

18.1 Elements of QbD

Four main elements of QbD are:

- Risk assessment approaches which begin with mapping tools such as flow-down map, process map, Ishikawa diagram to evaluate their knowledge space and further risk management tools such as failure modes and effects analysis (FMEA).
- PAT tools including in-process monitoring and multivariate systems.
- Mathematical and statistical tools which can be used in the planning, designing and analysing the experiment: statistical design of experiments (DoE).
- Continuous improvement tools which are implemented throughout process/product lifecycle to maintain the robust QbD construct.

18.2 Steps Involved in QbD Development Process

- Begin with a target product profile that describes the use, safety and efficacy of the product.
- Define a target product quality profile that will be used by formulators and process engineers as a quantitative surrogate for aspects of clinical safety and efficacy during product development.
- Gather relevant prior knowledge about the drug substance, potential excipients and process operations into a knowledge space. Use risk assessment to prioritize knowledge gaps for further investigation.
- Design a formulation and identify the critical material (quality) attributes of the final product that must be controlled to meet the target product quality profile.
- Design a manufacturing process to produce a final product having these critical material attributes.
- Identify the critical process parameters and input (raw) material attributes that must be controlled to achieve these critical material attributes of the final product. Use risk assessment to prioritize process parameters and material attributes for experimental verification. Combine prior knowledge with experiments to establish a design space or other representation of process understanding.

- Establish a control strategy for the entire process that may include input material controls, process controls and monitors, design spaces around individual or multiple unit operations, and/or final product tests. The control strategy should encompass expected changes in scale and can be guided by a risk assessment.
- Continually monitor and update the process to assure consistent quality.

18.3 The Principle Steps in QbD are:

- **Quality Target Product Profile (QTPP):** A prospective summary of the quality characteristics of a drug product that ideally will be achieved to ensure the desired quality, taking into account safety and efficacy of the drug product.

  It relates to quality, safety and efficacy, considering e.g., the route of administration, dosage form, bioavailability, strength, closure container system, therapeutic moiety release and stability.
- **Critical Quality Attribute (CQA):** A physical, chemical, biological, or microbiological property or characteristic that should be within an appropriate limit, range, or distribution to ensure the desired product quality.
- **Control Strategy:** A planned set of controls, derived from current product and process understanding that ensures process performance and product quality. The controls can include parameters and attributes related to drug substance and drug product materials and components, facility and equipment operating conditions, in-process controls, finished product specifications, and the associated methods and frequency of monitoring and control.
- **Critical Process Parameter (CPP):** A process parameter whose variability has an impact on a critical quality attribute and therefore should be monitored or controlled to ensure the process produces the desired quality.
- **Design Space:** The relationship between the process inputs (material attributes and process parameters) and the critical quality attributes can be described in the design space. Selection of variables, Describing a design Space in a submission, Unit operation design space, Relationship of

design space to scale and equipment, Design space versus proven acceptable ranges, Design space and edge of failure.

- **Continuous Improvements:** Process performance can be monitored to ensure that it is working as anticipated to deliver product quality attributes as predicted by the design space. This monitoring could include trend analysis of the manufacturing process as additional experience is gained during routine manufacture.

18.4 QbD Documents

- **Risk Assessment Report(s):** Performed throughout QbD Process and Particularly important to process development.
- **Quality Target Product Profile (QTPP):** Defines the desired product characteristics and sets development goals.
- **Control Strategy Summary:** Defines the process, its inputs and outputs, and how it is controlled.
- **PPQ Report(s):** Formal verification that the process Control Strategy has been defined appropriately and repeatedly produces the desired results.
- **Continued Process Verification (CPV) Reports:** Assuring that during routine commercial production, the process remains in a state **of control (FDA); involves feedback loops into the QbD "process" where intentional** process changes and/or observed variability is assessed for risk, characterized, re-validated, etc.

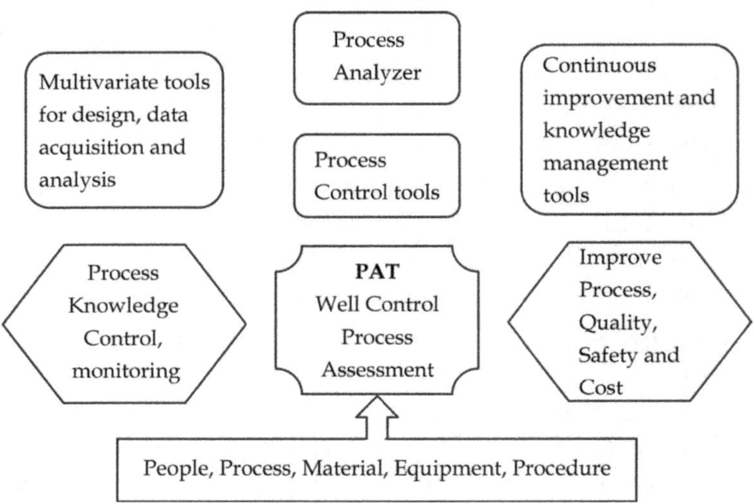

18.5 Process Analytical Technology (PAT) Frame Work

Before starting PAT one should answer following questions

- Why do PAT
- When to Apply
- Who benefits?
- Where does PAT begin and end?
- What to do with data?
- How to apply?
- Is the PAT for Process Knowledge or Process Control?

18.6 Use of PAT Tools in Continuous Manufacturing Process

There are many tools available that enables process understanding for scientific, risk-managed pharmaceutical Development, manufacture, and quality assurance. These tools, when used within a system, can provide effective and efficient means for acquiring information to facilitate process understanding, continuous improvement, and development of risk-mitigation strategies.

A. **PAT Tools:**

- Multivariate tools for design, data acquisition and analysis,
- Process analyzers,
- Process control tools,
- Continuous improvement and knowledge management tools.

B. **Risk-Based Approach:** Within an established quality system and for a particular manufacturing process, one would expect an inverse relationship between the level of process understanding and the risk of producing a poor quality product. For processes that are well understood, opportunities exist to develop less restrictive regulatory approaches to manage change. Thus, a focus on process understanding can facilitate risk-based regulatory decisions and innovation.

C. **Integrated Systems Approach:** Bringing the development, manufacturing, QA, and information/knowledge management functions so closely together that these four areas should be coordinated in an integrated manner.

D. **Real Time Release:** Real time release is the ability to evaluate and ensure the acceptable quality of in-process and/or final product based on process data. Typically, the PAT component of real time release includes a valid **combination of assessed material attributes and process controls.**

E. **Strategy for Implementation:** PAT principles & tools should be introduced during the development phase. When using new measurement tools, such as on- or in-line process analyzers, certain data trends, intrinsic to a currently acceptable process, may be observed. Manufacturers should scientifically evaluate these data to determine how or if such trends affect quality and implementation of PAT tools.

F. **Pat Regulatory Approach:**

- Improve the scientific basis for establishing regulatory specifications,
- Promote continuous improvement,
- Improve manufacturing while maintaining or improving the current level of product quality PAT implementation plans should be risk based. PAT can be implemented under the facility's own quality system. PAT implementation plans neither affect the current process nor require a change in specifications.

18.7 Product Life Cycle

"Product life cycle means all phases in the life of a product from the initial development through marketing until the product's discontinuation".

Product and process knowledge should be managed from development through the commercial life of the product up to and including product discontinuation. Sources of knowledge include, but are not limited to prior knowledge, pharmaceutical development studies; technology transfer activities; process validation studies over the product lifecycle; manufacturing experience; innovation; continual improvement; and change management activities.

The product lifecycle includes the following technical activities for new and existing products:

A. **Pharmaceutical Development:**
- Drug substance development;
- Formulation development (including container/ closure system);
- Manufacture of investigational products;
- Delivery system development (where relevant);
- Manufacturing process development and scale-up;
- Analytical method development.

B. **Technology Transfer:**
- New product transfers during Development through Manufacturing;
- Transfers within or between manufacturing and testing sites for marketed products.

C. **Commercial Manufacturing:**
- Acquisition and control of materials;
- Provision of facilities, utilities, and equipment;
- Production (including packaging and labelling);
- Quality control and assurance;
- Release;
- Storage;
- Distribution (excluding wholesaler activities).

D. **Product Discontinuation:**
- Retention of documentation;
- Sample retention;
- Continued product assessment and reporting.

The implementation of QbD requires appropriate PAT to monitor CQAs and CPPs during the processing of pharmaceuticals products to ensure that the product meets the desired quality attributes and reduce the risk of the poor manufacturing process performance and substandard pharmaceutical reaching patient. Risk is minimized by reducing variations in the process, while accuracy, repeatability and reproducibility are increased. There is no signal way of implementing QbD in practices. The ICH guidance documents lay the ground work for a better understanding on how to achieve QbD and improve product and process understanding.

18.8 Definition

- **Capability of a Process:** Ability of a process to realize a product that will fulfil the requirements of that product. The concept of process capability can also be defined in statistical terms. (ISO 9000:2005)
- **Continual Improvement:** Recurring activity to increase the ability to fulfil requirements. (ISO 9000:2005)
- **Control Strategy:** A planned set of controls, derived from current product and process understanding, that assures process performance and product quality. The controls can include parameters and attributes related to drug substance and drug product materials and components, facility and equipment operating conditions, in-process controls, finished product specifications, and the associated methods and frequency of monitoring and control.
- **Design Space:** The multidimensional combination and interaction of input variables (e.g., material attributes) and process parameters that have been demonstrated to provide assurance of quality.
- **Enabler:** A tool or process which provides the means to achieve an objective.
- **Knowledge Management:** Systematic approach to acquiring, analyzing, storing, and disseminating information related to products, manufacturing processes and components.

- **State of Control:** A condition in which the set of controls consistently provides assurance of continued process performance and product quality.
- **Proven Acceptable Range:** A characterized range of a process parameter for which operation within this range, while keeping other parameters constant, will result in producing a material meeting relevant quality criteria.

CHAPTER 19

Process Validation in Pharmaceutical Industry

Introduction

- Process validation is documented evidence that the process, operated within established parameters, can perform effectively and reproducibly to produce a medicinal product meeting its predetermined specifications and quality attributes. Process validation confirm that the control strategy are adequate to the process design and the quality of the product. A successful process validation program depends upon information and knowledge from product and process development. Process validation incorporates a lifecycle approach linking product and process development, validation of the commercial manufacturing process and maintenance of the process in a state of control during routine commercial production.

  Main component of process validation is process characterization and process verification.
- Process characterization consists of process development and process evaluation to ensure product and process is adequately designed.
- Process verification confirm that the final established manufacturing process is based on the process evaluation studies performs effectively in routine manufacture and is able to produce an active substance or intermediate or finished product of the desired quality on an appropriate number of consecutive batches produced with the commercial process and scale.

  The number of process validation batches depends on several factors including, but not limited to: (1) the complexity of the process being validated; (2) the level of process variability;

(3) the amount of experimental data and/or process knowledge available on the process; and (4) the frequency and cause(s) of deviations and batch failure.

Process validation should not be viewed as a one-time event. Process validation incorporates a lifecycle approach linking product and process development, validation of the commercial manufacturing process and maintenance of the process in a state of control during routine commercial production.

19.1 Approach of Process Validation

"Process validation is defined as the collection and evaluation of data, from the process design stage through commercial production, which establishes scientific evidence that a process is capable of consistently delivering quality product throughout its life cycle."

Process validation. Approach consists of following three stage.

A. **Stage 1 - Process Design:** Based on knowledge gained through development and scale-up activities.

B. **Stage 2 - Process Qualification:** During this stage, the process design is evaluated to determine if the process is capable of reproducible commercial manufacturing.

C. **Stage 3 - Continued Process Verification:** Ongoing assurance is gained during routine production that the process remains in a state of control.

A. **Stage 1 - Process Design:**

This stage helps to design and understand process attributes by Design of Experiment (DOE) in development stage. Process knowledge gain for each unit operation from the DOE will reduce number. The results of DOE studies provide justification for establishing ranges of incoming component quality, equipment parameters and in process quality attributes. All DOE and outcome must be document. This information is useful during the process qualification and continued process verification stages, including when the design is revised or the strategy for control is refined or changed.

B. Stage 2 - Process Qualification:

Process qualification confirms reproducibility of process during its commercial production by evaluation of process control parameters established during process design phase.

- Facility, Utilities and equipment must be qualified and documented with conclusion in the reports. Proper designing of the facility, Selecting utilities and equipment construction materials, operating principles, and play important role in process qualification.
- Process performance qualification is the combination of qualified facility, utilities, equipment, and the trained personnel with the commercial manufacturing process, control procedures, and components to produce commercial batches. It is one of the important milestone in product life cycle and must be completed before commercial distribution of product. The approach of PPQ must be depends on prior knowledge from process design and scientifically sound at every manufacturing unit process stage. During PPQ sampling and testing plan must be defined at higher level to have of great scrutiny and monitoring the process performance at every process stage .The process design stage and the process qualification stage must focus on the measurement system and control loop for the measured attribute.
- PPQ protocol must approved and contents details such as; the manufacturing conditions including operating parameters, processing limits, and component (raw material) inputs, sampling, test to be performed, Design of facilities and the qualification of utilities and equipment, personnel training and qualification, and verification of material source, Status of the validation of analytical methods used in measuring the process, inprocess materials, and the product and expected outcomes is essential for this stage of process validation.
- PPQ report must consist details such as; summarization of all activities carried with evaluation of testing parameters, unexpected observations, non-conformance observation, change control and state a clear conclusion as to whether the data indicates the process met the conditions

established in the protocol and whether the process is considered to be in a state of control. If not, the report should state what should be accomplished before such a conclusion can be reached. This conclusion should be based on a documented justification for the approval of the process, and release of lots produced by it to the market in consideration of the entire compilation of knowledge and information gained from the design stage through the process qualification stage.

C. Stage 3 – Continued Process Verification:

CPV is the ongoing program to verify and assessment critical quality attribute (CQA) and critical process parameter (CPP) to demonstrate that a process that operates within the predefined specified parameters consistently produces material which meets all its critical quality attributes (CQAs) and control strategy requirements. The data collected during review period is statistically trended and reviewed by trained personnel. Continuous process verification can be introduced at any time in the lifecycle of the product. It can be used for the initial commercial production, to re-validate commercialized products as part of process changes or to support continual improvement.

D. Revalidation:

Revalidation is necessary to ensure that the intentional or unintentional changes, in the production process, equipment and in the environment, do not affect adversely the characteristics of the process and the product quality. Revalidation can be divided in two broad categories:

- Revalidation after any change that may alter the product quality including transfer of processes from one company to another or from one site to another.
- Periodic revalidation carried out at scheduled intervals , which are justified:

19.2 Content of Validation Protocol/Report

A written approved protocol and report must be available before product available.

- Product Name.

- Objectives.
- Scope.
- Justification for Validation.
- Validation team.
- Responsibilities of Validation team.
- Risk Assessment.
- Type of validation: Prospective, concurrent, Retrospective, revalidation.
- Number of batches to be validated.
- Controls: Approved mater formula, standard operating procedure and methods, qualification, requalification and preventive maintenance of equipment used.
- Critical process parameters and their respective tolerance.
- Description of the processing steps: copy of the master documents for the product.
- Sampling points: Stages of sampling, methods of sampling and sampling plans.
- Statistical tools to be used in the analysis of data.
- Forms and chart to be used for documenting results.
- Non-conference (Out of Specification/Out of Trend/ Deviation).
- Change control.
- Conclusion.
- Summary.
- Approval of study.
- The validation protocol Report should be numbered, signed and dated.

CHAPTER 20

Cleaning Validation and Cross Contamination Approach on Risk MaPP Concept

Introduction

Cleaning validation plays an important role in reducing the possibility of product contamination by consistently removes product residues, process residues and environmental contaminants from the manufacturing equipment/system, so that this equipment/system can be safely used for the manufacture same or a different product.

Cleaning process requires multiple steps such as cleaning cycle, use and type of detergents and/or solvent, presence of an acid cleaning, concentration of cleaning agents, contact time of cleaning agents on equipment, feed pressure or flow rate, cleaning temperature, and required length or volume, length and/or number of rinse step. During designing cleaning validation program physical aspects shall be followed commonly known as "TACT".

- **Time:** Defined the length of time for the cycle step.
- **Action:** Mechanism used to deliver the cleaning agent
- **Cleaning agent:** Concentrations directly affect the performance of the cleaning process, easily removed.
- **Optimal temperature Ranges:** Will vary for the different steps of the cleaning process.

20.1 Types of Cleaning

Cleaning of the equipment can be done in three Ways Manual, Semi Auto and Automatic Cleaning of Equipment. In cleaning, Standard operating procedure pays an important role. Standard procedure should be clear to follow the steps for operator: Dissemble, assemble, difficult to clean areas, feasibility, the procedure should reproducibility and operator training.

A. **Manual Cleaning** is defined as the direct cleaning of equipment by a trained equipment operator using a variety of hand tools and cleaning agents. Important cleaning parameters for manual cleaning may include : Volume of cleaning agents ,Volume of rinse water, Temperature of wash and rinse solutions, Sequence and duration (contact time) of soaking, wash and rinse steps, Scrubbing action, Pressure of solutions and Detergent concentration.

B. **Semi-Automated Processes Cleaning:** Cleaning is intermediate between fully automated and fully manual cleaning. During the automatic cleaning gasket fitting, Assembly fitting consist manual cleaning and then automatic cleaning.

C. **Automated Processes Cleaning:** APC is controlled by program through relay logic, a computer or programmable logic controller (PLC).The control system regulates the cleaning cycles, addition of cleaning agents, temperature, time and other critical cleaning parameters. Important cleaning parameters for automated cleaning may include the volume of cleaning agents, volume of rinse water, flow rates and temperature of wash and rinse solutions, duration of wash and rinse cycles, pressure of solution, operating ranges and detergent concentration.

20.2 Approach for Cleaning Validation

Pharmaceutical industry follows mainly two approaches for cleaning validation: Product grouping and Equipment Grouping.

- Products may be grouped together if they are manufactured on the same or equivalent equipment and cleaned by the same cleaning procedure.
- Equipment may be grouped together if they are similar and can be cleaned by the same cleaning procedure. The grouping strategy is based on designating equipment as "identical" or "similar," based on design, **mode of operation, and clean ability.**

20.3 Addition of New Product and Equipment to Validated Chain

- The introduction of a new product into an already validated group is assessed using the same science and risk-based evaluation process (e.g., based on solubility in the cleaning solvent, a laboratory coupon study, and/or information from other process cleaning studies) to initially determine the worst-case product. It is recommended that if each new product is tested in a lab evaluation, a suitable control, such as the previous worst-case product, be included.
- The introduction of new similar equipment requires an evaluation if that new equipment represents a new worst case or a new bracketing extreme. If not a new worst case or new extreme, special attention should be paid to the first commercial cleaning event to confirm effectiveness. If the new equipment is a new worst case or bracketing extreme, the validation requirements for the previous worst case or bracketing extreme should be performed for the new worst-case or bracketing extreme equipment.

20.4 Equipment Hold Study Approaches

- *Dirty Hold Time*: Dirty hold time for equipment is time between completion of use and initiation of cleaning. Dirty hold time shall be clearly justified and documented in protocol
- *Clean Hold Time*: Equipment time between completion of cleaning and next use.
- *Campaign Cleaning Validation*: Campaign is a series of batches of the same product manufactured equipment. Campaign run on equipment can impact the cleaning validation programs due to prolong material contact with equipment or environment impact. To prove no impact on campaign run cleaning validation shall be performed of defined tome period and number or batches taken on campaign. Based on validation campaign length needs to be defined.

20.5 Selection of Worst Case Product

- *Therapeutic Class*: Therapeutic class shall be considered for the selection of molecules.

- *Drug Potency*: The Drug having highest potency shall be considered for the selection. Within the selected molecule of having various strength the drug with highest strength shall be considered.
- *Solubility*: The drug with least solubility in water shall be considered for the selection.
- *Specific Method of Cleaning*: Product involving use of specific cleaning method or use of cleaning agent cleaning agent shall be considered.

20.6 Cleaning Validation Protocol

Cleaning validation protocol should consist: Objective, Purpose, Scope, Responsibility, Reason for validation, Cleaning and Sampling procedure, Testing procedure, Bioburden Limits, Acceptance criteria, Deviations, Revalidation.

- Bioburdenlimit in cleaning validation shall be established, limits can be established using carryover calculations. Typical bioburden limits for non-sterile manufacturing (1-2 CFU/cm2) is considered more than adequate for surface sampling. For rinse sampling that is performed with WFI, one approach is to utilize typical WFI values (10 CFU/100 mL), while another approach is to utilize a value of either 100 CFU/100 mL or 1,000 CFU/100 mL.
- *Visual Inspection*: Visual appearance of production surfaces is a direct measurement that verifies removal of residuals. The use of optical equipment like mirrors or endoscopes, use of additional lighting, can be used for visual inspection.
- *Sampling Method Selection*: **Selection** of a sampling method depends on the nature of the equipment, the nature of the residue being measured, the residue limit, and the desired analytical method.

A. **Indirect Sampling: Rinse Sampling:** Rinse sampling involves sampling the equipment by flowing solvent over all relevant equipment surfaces to remove residues, which are then measured in the rinse solvent. Collection of rinse samples should consider solubility, location, timing and volume.

B. **Direct Sampling: Swab Sampling:** Swabbing involves wiping a surface with fibrous material which non-shredded, no extractable, no interference with sample and flexible.

- ***Sampling Recovery Studies*:** Sampling recovery studies are generally required to adequately demonstrate that a residue, if present on equipment surfaces, can be adequately measured or quantified by the combination of the analytical method and the sampling procedure. Sampling recovery studies are laboratory studies involving coupons of sampled equipment of different materials of construction (such as stainless steel, glass, PTFE, and EPDM) spiked with residues to be measured.
- Methods of Calculating Acceptance Criteria:

A. **Toxicological Data:** Therapeutic dose is not know

$NOEL = LD_{50}(g/kg) \times 70(Kg\ per\ person / 2000)$

$MACO = NOAEL \times MBS / Safety\ factor \times TDD_{next}$

B. **Therapeutic Daily Dose:** no greater than 1/1000 of the normal Therapeutic dose will be present per typical dose of the next product to be run in the equipment.

$MACO = TDD_{previous} \times MBS / Safety\ factor \times TDD_{next}$

C. **10ppm criteria 10ppm:** up to 0.1% in next product (Based on the ICH impurity document which indicates that up to 0.1% of an individual unknown or 0.5%.

$MACO_{ppm} = MAXCONC \times 0.001\%\ MBS$

$CONC = MACO/MBS$

D. ***General Criteria Rinse & Swab*: Surface area and Volume is known**

Swab Limit = MACO /Surface Area

Rinse Limit =MACO/ Volume

Safety Factor

Topical 10 - 100

Oral product 100 - 1000

Parenteral 1000 - 10000

- **MBS** : Minimum batch size for the next product(s)
- **SF :** Safety factor
- **TDDnext**Largest normal daily dose for the next product
- **MACO :** Maximum Allowable Carryover
- **NOEL :** No Observed Effect Level
- 2000 : is an empirical constant
- **70 kg :** is the weight of an average adult
- **MAXCONC:** maximum allowed con centration (kg/kg or ppm) of "previous" substance in the next batch.

20.7 Quality Risk based Approach for Cleaning Validation

- Risk of cross-contamination can be evaluated by toxicity, quantity of active used per batch, process train used in product manufacture, level of containment, the use of shared equipment, opportunity to contaminate, dosing regimen of the product, daily doses contained in a batch, frequency of the ingredient's or product's.
- Risk based should be based on approach holistic review by considering multi-disciplinary task depends on knowledge of product, process, challenge and question ask to process. Risk base approach to the cleaning validation shall be depends on toxicology, hygienist, engineers, quality mangers, users or operating personnel and independent facilitator.

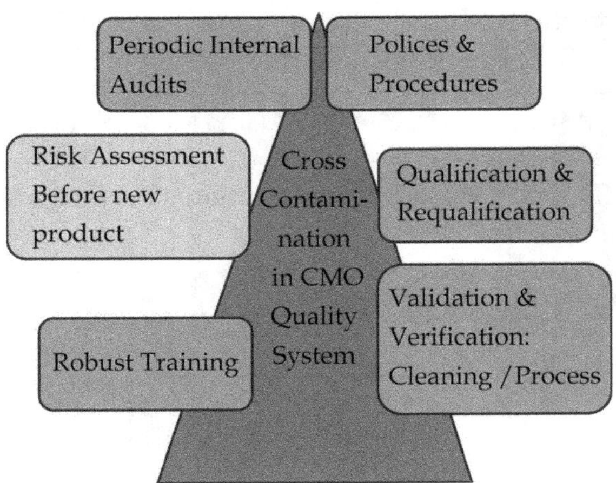

Regulatory requirements Risk Map Concept

- Recently regulatory agency challenge to develop an approach for managing risk at its multiproduct facility, different active pharmaceutical ingredients, including high potency APIs (HAPIs).

- Risk-MaPP-Q9 approach is designed to identify and focus on critical risk areas.
- Risk assessment tool allows to assign a numeric value, not only to each potential source of cross-Contamination risk, but also to products that are vulnerable to cross- Contamination.

20.8 European Union Expectation on Cross Contamination

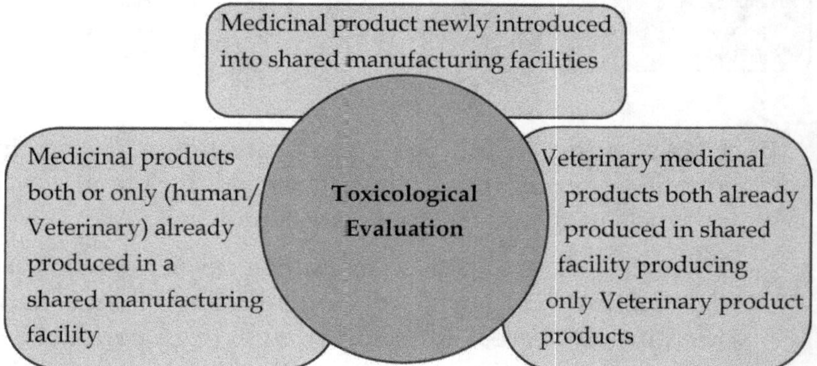

Prevention of cross-contamination should be based on the **toxicological evaluation** (Figure 2). From the toxicological Evaluation and risk identification dedicated facilities requirement shall be decided. Risk in manufacturing of medicinal product may be because of:

- The risk cannot be adequately controlled by operational and/ or technical measures,
- Scientific data from the toxicological evaluation does not support a controllable risk (e.g. allergenic potential from highly sensitizing materials such as beta lactams) or
- Relevant residue limits, derived from the toxicological evaluation, cannot be satisfactorily determined by a validated analytical method.

A. **EU Chapter 5 Expectation:** The QRM process shall periodically reviewed for effectiveness. (Figure 3 & 4). Evaluation to be assess and Control the cross-contamination during manufacturing product which are based on **technical and organizational measures.**

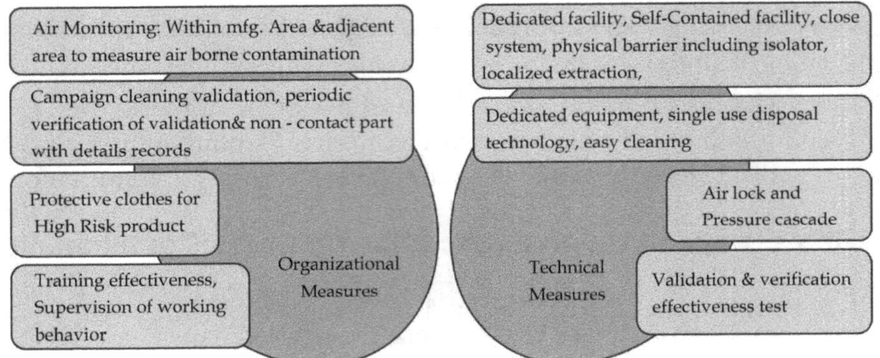

B. EMA: Setting Health Based Exposure Limits for use in risk identification in the manufacture of different medicinal products in shared facilities Expectation:

To review & evaluate pharmacological & toxological data (non-clinical & clinical) of individual API and derive a scientifically based threshold value (e.g. permitted daily exposure (PDE-(Figure 25) or threshold of toxicological concern (TTC) for individual active substances.

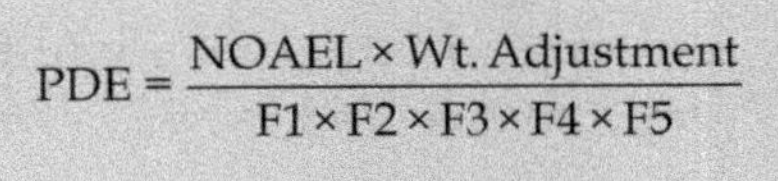

$$PDE = \frac{NOAEL \times Wt.\ Adjustment}{F1 \times F2 \times F3 \times F4 \times F5}$$

The PDE represents a substance-specific dose that is unlikely to cause an adverse effect if an individual is exposed at or below this dose every day for a lifetime. Determination of a PDE involves:

- Hazard identification by reviewing all relevant data,
- Identification of "critical effects",
- Determination of the NOAEL of the findings that are considered to be critical effects, and
- Use of several adjustment factors (F1 to F5) to account for various uncertainties
- F1: A factor (values between 2 and 12) to account for extrapolation between species, F2: A factor of 10 to account for variability between individuals, F3: A factor 10 to account for repeat-dose toxicity studies of short duration, i.e., less than 4-weeks ,F4: A factor (1-10) that may be applied in cases of severe toxicity, e.g. non-genotoxic carcinogenicity, neurotoxicity or teratogenicity,

F5: A variable factor that may be applied if the no-effect level was not established. When only an LOEL is available, a factor of up to 10 could be used depending on the severity of the toxicity.

20.9 Selection & Reporting of the PDE Determination Strategy

- Appropriate PDE to be used for the cleaning validation process should be made with an appropriate justification. Usually, by default the lowest PDE value will be used.
- The identification of a "critical effect should be based on a comprehensive literature and reviewed by expert with clear rationale on the adjustment factors that were applied in deriving the PDE. The initial page of any prepared PDE determination strategy document should be a summary of the assessment process.

20.10 Non-Penicillin Beta-Lactam Drugs: A CGMP Framework for Preventing Cross-Contamination

- Separate and isolated operation facility (manufacture, processing, and packing) for pencilline. Additionally, requires to test non-penicillin drug products for penicillin where the possibility of exposure to cross-contamination exists, and prohibits manufacturers from marketing such products if detectable levels of penicillin are found.

20.11 Definitions

- *Clean*: Having product residues, process residues, and environmental contaminants removed to an acceptable level.
- *Cleaning Validation*: Documented evidence with a high degree of assurance that a cleaning process will result in products meeting their predetermined quality attributes throughout its life cycle.
- *Cleaning Verification*: A one-time sampling and testing to ensure that specified equipment has been properly cleaned following a specific cleaning event.
- *Cleaning Procedure*: The documentation that assures any product and process-related material introduced into

equipment as part of the manufacturing process stream is removed and the equipment is adequately stored.

- ***Cleaning Agent***: The solution or solvent used in the washing step of a cleaning process. Examples of cleaning agents are water, organic solvent, commodity chemical diluted in water, and formulated detergent diluted in water.
- ***Contamination***: An undesired residue or residue level on cleaned equipment surfaces or in a manufactured product.
- ***Clean Hold Time***: The time from the end of the cleaning process until the equipment is used again (which may be product manufacture, autoclaving, or a steam in-place (SIP) cycle).
- ***Dirty Hold Time***: The time from the end of product manufacturing until the beginning of the cleaning process (also called "soiled hold time").
- ***Equipment Train***: The sequence of equipment through which a product is produced or processed.
- ***Grouping Strategy***: A strategy for establishing similar cleaning processes, usually based on similar products or similar equipment, and to validate the cleaning process based primarily on validation data for a representative of the group.
- ***Recovery Study***: A laboratory study combining the sampling method and analytical method to determine the quantitative recovery of a specific residue for a defined surface.
- ***Residue***: Chemical or microbiological material remaining on equipment surfaces after a cleaning process.
- ***Worst-Case Process Condition***: A condition or set of conditions encompassing upper and/or lower processing limits and circumstances, within standard operating procedures, which pose the greatest chance of product or process failure when compared to ideal conditions (such conditions do not necessarily induce product or process failure).
- ***Worst Case Soil:*** A soil that is the most difficult to clean from production equipment based on knowledge generated from laboratory studies, scientific properties, and/or production experience.

- *Campaign*: Processing of multiple lots or batches of the same product serially in the same equipment.
- *Changeover*: The steps taken for switching multiproduct equipment from the manufacture of one product to the manufacture of a different product.
- *Acceptable Daily Exposure*: A dose that is unlikely to cause an adverse effect if an individual is exposed, by any route, at or below this dose every day for a lifetime.
- *Acceptable Daily Intake*: An amount of a substance consumed on a daily basis that is considered at a safe level.
- *Acceptance Criteria*: Numerical limits, ranges, or other suitable measures for the acceptance of test results.
- *Acceptance Limit*: The maximum amount of residue allowed in a product, in an analytical sample, or as an amount per surface area.

CHAPTER 21

Pharmaceutical Water Generation and Distribution System and Regulatory Expectation

Introduction

Water is one of the major commodities used by the pharmaceutical industry. It may be used as an excipient, or used for reconstitution of product, during synthesis, during production of the finished product or as a cleaning agent for rinsing vessels, equipment, primary packing material etc. Different grades of water quality are required depending on the different pharmaceutical uses.

- Validation and qualification of water purification, storage and distribution system are a fundamental part of GMP and form an integral part of GMP inspection.

21.1 Design and Process Flow

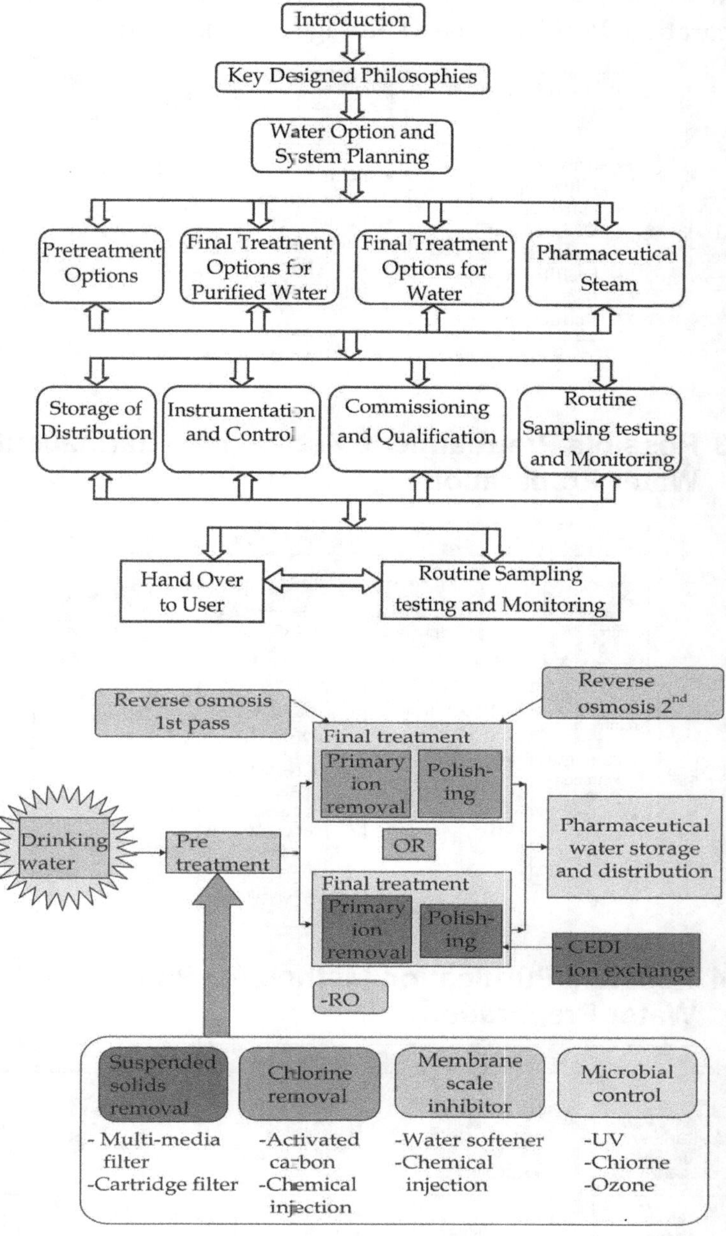

General Steps in pharmaceutical Water System

21.2 Steps involved in Pharmaceutical Water Preparations

Mainly Pharmaceutical Water Preparation consist below three steps: Preparation, Purification and Storage and distribution.

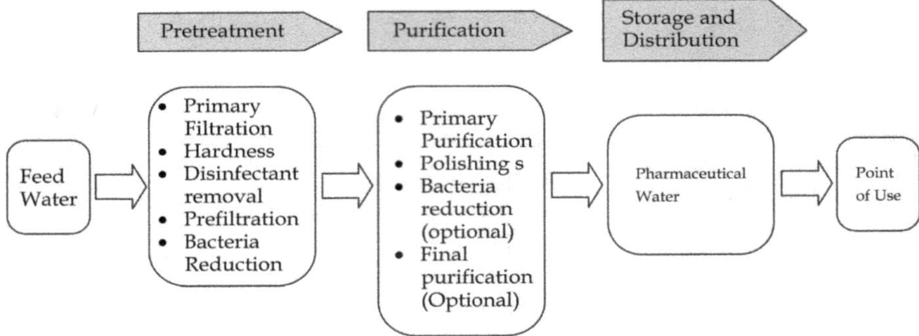

21.3 Possible Pretreatment Method for Pharmaceutical Water Preparation

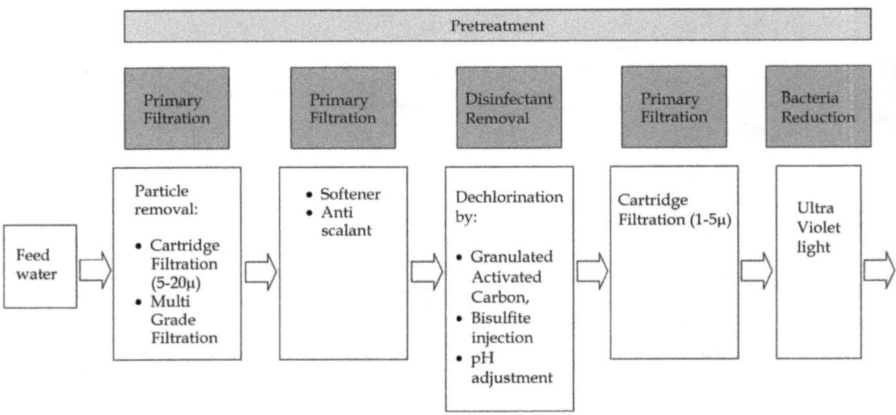

21.4 Possible Purification Method for Pharmaceutical Water Preparation

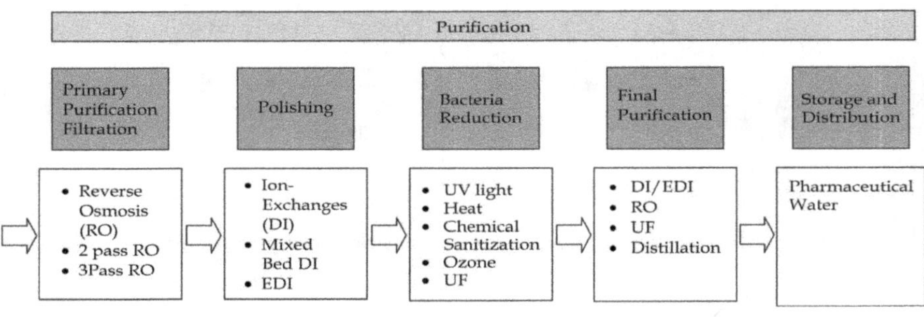

21.5 Qualification

A. **User Requirement Specification (URS):** The URS is developed during the conceptual design phase and should be reviewed and updated throughout the life cycle of the project. URS review results shall be summarized in report.

a. **Process water:** Process water delivered to points of use, shall meets the quality specification for US EPA or IS 10500 drinking water or appropriate national drinking water specifications. Additionally, no coliforms shall be present. Microbial colony forming level shall less than 500 cfu's/ml.

b. **Purified water/water for injection:** Purified water and WFI generation train shall meet the respective water specification.

c. **Pure steam:**

- Pure steam from the generator, upon condensation, shall meet the same chemical and Endotoxin quality specification as WFI.
- Pure steam from the generator shall have-a dryness value of not less than 0.9 for porous loads for autoclaving, a dryness value of not less than 0.95 for metal loads for autoclaving, superheat content, which does not exceed 25oC and non-condensable gas not exceeding 3.5% by volume. Some steam applications not require non-condensable gas limits

B. **Functional Design Specification (FDS):**

- The FDS are tested or verified during commissioning or OQ. The FDS shall include requirements such as:
- Specific capacity and flow of the water system.
- High purity water generation system feed water quality
- Alarms and message
- Point of use, water flow, temperature and pressure
- Sanitization techniques to be used for the storage and distribution system
- General human/Machine interface(HMI)layout
- Process control system strategy including input/output and interlock configurations
- Electronic data storage and system security.

a. **Process water:**

- Process water pumps shall be able to deliver 3.05kg/sq.cm (100ft) of head, while delivering 380L/min (100gpm) to the piping and point to use network.
- The free chlorine injection system shall provide maintenance of 0.5 ppm of free chlorine in the flowing process water distribution system.
- Main distribution and branch and branch piping shall achieve a "flush to drain" water of 1.5 m/sec (5ft/sec).

b. **Purified water /WFI:**

- Feed water to the purified water generation system shall be of US EPA Primary Drinking water Quality shall have< 500 ppm hardness(as CaCO3)
- In-line TOC and conductivity measurements shall be the primary method to monitor WFI quality compliance.
- Reynolds number in the re-circulation piping section of the distillation loop shall be sufficient for fully turbulent conditions at all times of system operation.
- Distribution system will be able to maintain water temperatures equal to or greater than 80oC at all times of operation.
- For the purified water distribution loop, system will be able to maintain ozone levels at 0.1 ppm in water in the storage vessel.
- The distribution loop shall be able to deliver 95 L/min (25gpm) at three points of use, while maintaining 2.8kg/sq.cm. (40 psig) at the spray nozzle inlet (return to vessel) during normal operation.
- The distribution system temperature control systems shall maintain.

c. **Pure steam:**

- The pure steam generator shall provide 454 kg/hr (1000 pounds/hr) of pure steam at 4.2 kg/sq.cm (60psi) at discharge of the generator using USP purified water feed water to the pure steam generator.
- Generator blow down shall be between 5% and 15% of generator capacity during normal operation.

C. Design Specification (DS):

DS specifies how to build the direct impact water or steam system. The DS is tested or verified during commissioning or IQ. The DS lists items for testing verification. The DS shall include items such as:

- Materials used to build the system that shall ensure continuous quality water or steam.
- Pump, heat exchanger, storage vessel, and other field device specifications, including critical instrument.
- Correct installation of equipment
- Documentation required for the system
- Storage vessel vent filter operation" (E.g. Electrical heat traces or steam heat traced)
- Treatment system description
- Electrical drawing
- Hardware specification.

a. Process water:

- Drawing or associated documentation for the process water distribution system shall include an "as-build" P & ID.
- The process water metal piping length shall be galvanized steel or equivalent inert material.
- Air gap's will be used to separate (provide back flow protection) process water points of use and drains.
- Distribution piping systems shall be designed without dead-ends (area of piping where the flow stops and cannot be drained).

b. Purified water /WFI:

- Piping, valves, pump wetted surfaces and other components that contact the WFI shall be manufactured from 316LSS and have a 20 RA finish.
- Slope of the pipeline shall be 1:100.
- Boroscope certificated for Welding joint.
- All branch valves, which separate branch piping from the main loop, will be connected to ensure compliance with the 6-D rule.

c. **Pure steam:**

- Provide sloping and slope map for the clean steam system.
- Pure steam piping distribution system shall be constructed of 316L SS.
- Steam traps are adequately installed to remove condensate.

D. **Performance Qualification for purified water / WFI / Pure Steam: Performance Qualification is done in three different phase:**

a. **Phase 1: Test period: 2–4 weeks:**

- During this period the system shall operate continuously without failure or performance deviation.
- Chemical and microbiological testing shall be performed in accordance with a defined plan to verify its quality.
- All sampling points should be covered in daily monitoring. Develop and finalize operating, cleaning, sanitizing and maintenance procedures.
- Verify provisional alert and action levels.
- Develop and refine test-failure procedure.
- Water cannot be used for manufacturing purpose during this phase.

b. **Phase 2: Test Period: 2–4 weeks:**

- The sampling schedule shall be generally the same as in phase 1.
- Water can be used for manufacturing purposes during this phase.
- Demonstrate the operation within established ranges.
- Demonstrate the delivery of water in accordance with the SOPs.

c. **Phase 3: Test Period: 1**

- Evaluation of seasonal variations.
- The sample locations, sampling frequencies and tests shall be reduced to the normal routine pattern based on established procedures proven during phases 1 and 2.

E. Validation Cycle of Qualification and Validation of Water System: (USP<1231>)

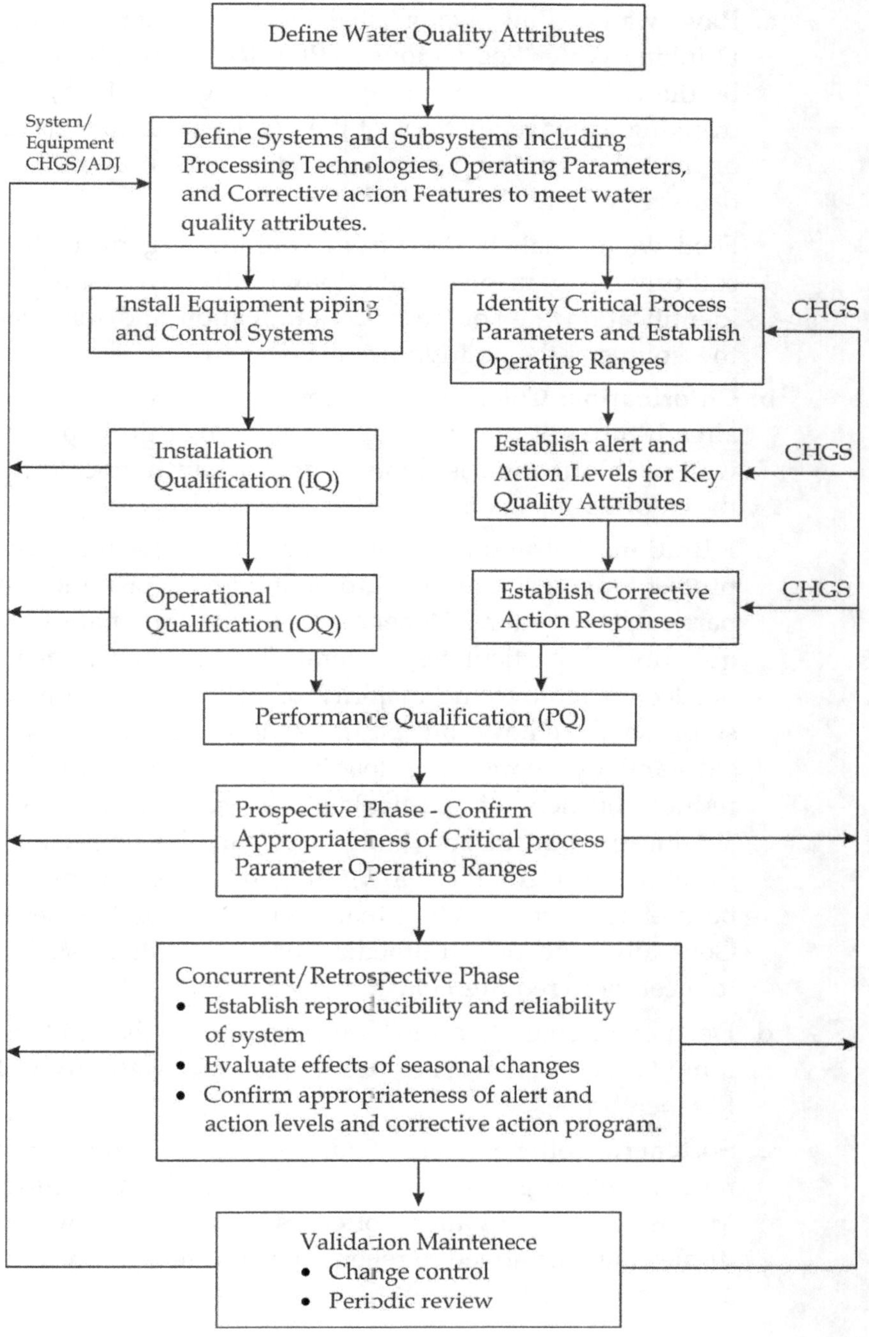

21.6 Component for Pharmaceutical Water System

A. Pretreatment System:

a. **Raw water:** Raw water shall meets National Primary Drinking Water Regulations (NPDWR) (40 CFR 141) issued by the U.S. Environmental Protection Agency (EPA) or the drinking water regulations of the European Union or Japan, or the WHO drinking water guideline and IS standard for drinking water.

   Feed water shall be free from coliform organism. If any coliform organisms are found the measures for identification the source of contamination and removal of the source of the pollution shall be taken.

b. **Chlorination:** Chlorination is done to inactivate organisms already present and to suppress microbial growth in raw water. Chlorination is done using sodium hypochlorite as the chlorinating agent.

c. **Filtration:** Filtration of raw water may be required to protect downstream equipment and process from particulate matter. Depending upon the nature and quantity of particulates, several filtration steps may be needed to remove the majority of particles .The filtration steps shall remove all particles above 50 microns and substantially reduce the loading of smaller particles to reduce burden of particulates in raw water. Where significant particulate build up can be expected on filtrations of incoming water, a regenerative system would be preferable to a system that utilizes disposable element. Generally sand or multimedia filtrations will be sufficient to meet these requirements.

d. **Dechlorination:** Sodium Metabisulphite is added to remove excess chlorine or ozone from raw water to protect RO membrane.

e. **Softener:** Softeners are Sodium-based cation-exchange resins. Softening is the removal of hardness (Calcium and Magnesium) from Water. Softeners are usually provided as duplex pairs arranged to regenerate at different times.

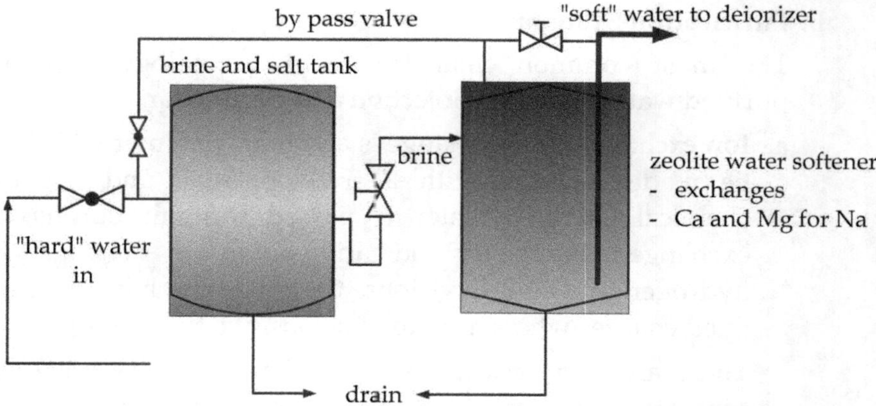

f. **Hardness:** Hardness measurements can be used to determine the Ca2– and Mg2+ concentrations before or after softening. The aim is to achieve a zero response after the softener, to protect downstream processes.

g. **Oxidation Reduction Potential (ORP):** Oxidation Reduction Potential also known as redox and is an electrochemical measurements of the ions in the water .OPR can be used during pretreatment to assess required pH adjustments or to measure chlorine, chloramine, bromine, and other oxidizing agents into single parameter for measurement.

h. **Silt density indicator:** Slit density indicator is commonly used to ensure the turbidity of water compliance with the (US) National Primary Drinking Water standards. The slit Density Index (SDI) test is used to determine the fouling potential of water feeding a membrane filtration process such as Reverse osmosis.

i. **Microbial-Retentive filtration:** Microbial retentive filters may be used downstream of unit operations that tend to release microorganisms or upstream of unit operations that are sensitive to microorganisms. Microbial retentive filters may also be used to filter water feeding the distribution system.

B. Purification System:

The most common final treatment technology used for purified water, water for injection and pure steam.

a. **Ion exchange:** Ion exchange is a organic polymer which can be made function with a fixed positive and negative chemical charges. Water is passed through porous ion exchange resign beads and cation-anion are exchanged for hydrogen and hydroxyl ions. Cation resins have negative fixed charges where as anion has positive fixed charges.

   There are two basic physical configuration: Two bed (or separate bed) dimineralizers regeneration system is divided in

   - ***Co-current*** regeneration system of two bed system: The regeneration fluid flows in the same direction of the process water stream.
   - ***Counter-current*** regeneration system of two bed system: The regeneration fluid flows in the opposite direction of the process water stream.

b. **Mixed bed dimineralizers:** Mixed bed demineralizers consist of a single tank with a mixture of cation and anion removal resin. The resins are thoroughly mixed in the service cycle and separate into two distinct layers for regeneration.

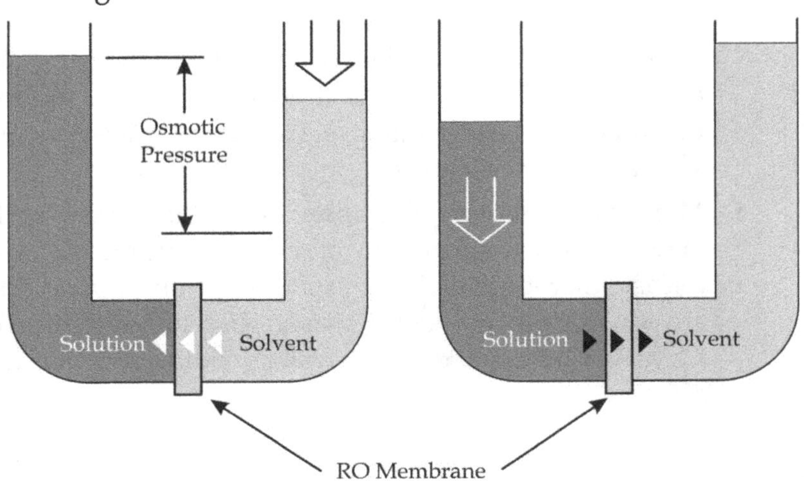

c. **Reserve osmosis:**

Reverse osmosis (RO) is a pressure driven process utilizing a semi-membrane capable of removing dissolved organic and inorganic contaminants from water. A semi permeable membrane is permeable to some substance such as water, while being impermeable to other substance, such as salts, acids, bases, colloidal, bacteria and endotoxins.

d. **Continuous electro deionization (CEDI) or Electron de-ionization (EDI):** Continuous Electrodeionization (CEDI) is a technology combining ion exchange resins, ion selective membranes and the use of an electrical field to continuously remove ionized species and regenerates resins. RO/CEDI systems can produce water with 0.1 µS/cm or lower conductivity.

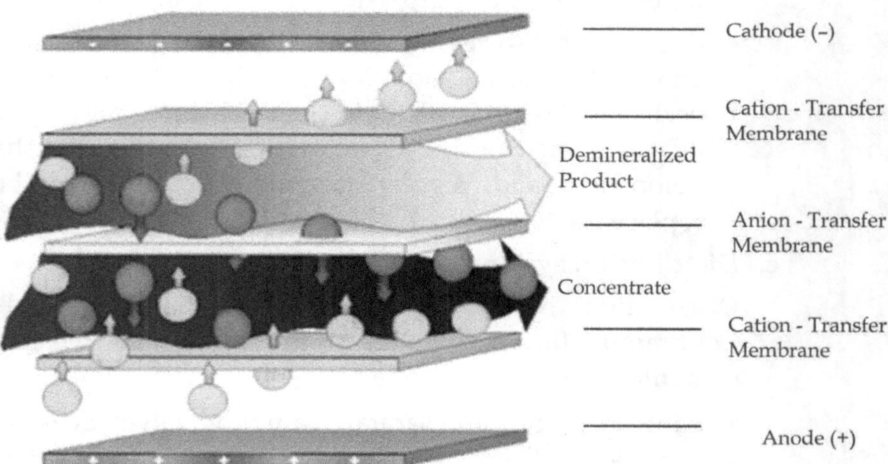

C. Storage and Distribution

a. **Storage tanks:** Storage tank shall be made of Material of construction SS316L, closed with smooth interiors and has the ability to spray the tank headspace using spray balls on recalculating loop returns, and the use of heated, jacketed/insulated tanks.

- Rupture disks is put on storage tank as safeguard. Jacketed Storage tank are to maintained the temperature.
- Hydrophobic microbial retentive membrane filter (vent filter) are affixed on storage tank for breathing.

- Vent filters integrity shall be tested in the housing prior to initial use, periodic and post integrity at the time the filter removed from service to assure that the preventive maintenance schedule and procedure are appropriate.
- Common filter integrity methods are bubble test, diffusion and water intrusion. Sanitization shall be performed as per validation and approved procedure.

b. Ultraviolet light: Ultraviolet radiation has widely been used as a germicidal treatment for water. Mercury low pressure lamps generating 254 nm UV light are an effective means of sanitizing water. The adsorption of UV light by the DNA and proteins in the microbial cell results in the inactivation of the microorganism.

- The combination of 186 and 254 wavelengths is necessary for the photo oxidation of organic compounds.
- Control measures include regular inspection or emissivity alarms to detect bulb failures or film occlusions, regular UV bulb sleeve cleaning and wiping, downstream chlorine detectors, downstream polishing deionizers, and regular (approximately yearly) bulb replacement.

c. Distribution systems:

Distribution system pipelines are made of SS316L. Continuous flow of water in the piping by means of recirculation is recommended

- Sanitary pumps and sanitary sampling valve are used in the system. Components and distribution lines shall be sloped and fitted with drain points so that the system can be completely drained (Normally 1:100).
- The distribution design shall include the placement of sampling valves in the storage tank and at other locations such as in the return line of the recirculating water system.
- One point in the distribution loop may be connected for preparation of Water for injection and Pure steam.
- Water for injection is produced by using Single Effect Distillation or Multiple Effect Distillation.

d. **Sanitization:** Systems can be sanitized using either thermal or chemical means.

  - Hot sanitization by water is done at least 80oC or by pure steam.
  - Ozone sanitization with limit NMT than 0.1 ppm in water in the storage vessel. Sanitization steps require validation to demonstrate the capability of reducing and holding microbial contamination at acceptable levels. The frequency of sanitization shall be established in such a way that the system operates in a state of microbiological control and does not routinely exceed alert limit. Sanitization shall be performed after replacement of pump, after calibration of equipment, break down or increase in bioload.

e. **Total Organic Carbon (TOC):** Total Organic Carbon is an indirect measure of organic compounds present in water and measured as carbon. Total Organic Carbon (TOC) is a sum measure of the concentration of all organic carbon atoms covalently bonded in the organic molecules of a given sample of water.

  - TOC is typically measured in Parts per Million (ppm or mg/L) or Parts per Billion (ppb or μg/L), or even Parts Per Trillion (ppt).

f. **Conductivity:** Conductivity measure non-specific conductive ions in the water. Temperature has a profound impact upon conductivity measurements because of the effect on ion mobilities.

g. **Flow of distribution loop:** Water flow rate (or velocity-fully turbulent Reynolds number) may help to reduce the microbiological growth and maintain temperature within hot or cold system. Sanitary flow sensors are recommended in distribution. Circulation at higher velocities help to maintain a uniform temperature throughout the distribution system loop of purified water and WFI pure steam condensate.

h. **Pressure:** Pressure in distribution system may be deemed critical to prevent leaks and avoid contamination due to backflow. Distribution loop return pressure may be important so as to develop vessel internal spray patterns.

i. **Micro filtration:** Microfiltration is a membrane process used for the removal of fine particles and microorganism. Microfiltration cartridge are disposable and ranges from 0.45 µm down to 0.04µm.

j. **Ultra filteration:** Membranes are made up of polymeric and ceramic materials. Polymeric membrane elements are available in spiral wound and hollow fiber configurations. Ceramic modules are available in single channel and multi channel configuration.

  - UF normally is used in still feed water system, in combination with ion exchange to limit the Endotoxin and colloidal silica feed levels.

k. **Pure steam:** Pure steam normally is generated in a shell and tube heat exchanger like evaporator. Feed water is introduced on the one side of the tubes, While the heating medium is introduced on the other side. Heating of the feed water is introduced on one side and boiling temperature causes the water to evaporate, producing steam. Typically pure steam pressure is 30 PSIG to 60 PSIG (2 BARG to 4 BARG)

21.7 Methods used for Preparation of Pharmaceutical Water

Type of Water	IP	USP	EP	BP
Drinking/ Potable water	As per National Requirement	As per National Requirement	As per National Requirement	As per National Requirement
Purified	Distillation/Ion exchange	De-ionization, distillation, ion exchange, RO	De-ionization, distillation, ion exchange, RO	De-ionization, distillation, ion exchange, RO
Highly Purified	NA	NA	NA	Double pass RO coupled with UF/Deionization
WFI	Distillation (Discard first portion)	Distillation/ RO	Distillation RO	Distillation

21.8 Test Performed for Potable Water and its Recommended Limits

- Hardness not more than 500 ppm.
- Coliform should be absent. If any coliform organisms are found the measures for identification the source of contamination and removal of the source of the pollution shall be taken.
- Microbial Monitoring NMT 500cfu per /ml.
- pH 5.0-7.0
- Residue on evaporation NMT 0.01%
- Periodic testing for Pesticides, Radio active substances, Organic or in organic compound as per IS 10500.

21.9 Type of water is used in the Pharmaceutical Sterile Medicine Product as an Excipient as per EMEA / CVMP / 115 / 01 Note for Guidance on Quality of Water for Pharmaceutical Use

Sr. No	Sterile Medicine product	Minimum Acceptable Quality of Water
1	Parental	Water for Injection
2	Ophthalmic	Purified Water
3	Haemo filteration Solution	Water for Injection
4	Peritoneal Dialysis Solution	Water for Injection
5	Irrigation Solution	Water for Injection
6	Nasal/Ear Preparations	Purified Water
7	Cutaneous Preparations	Purified Water

21.10 Type of water is used in the Pharmaceutical Non-Sterile Medicine Product as an Excipient as per EMEA / CVMP / 115 / 01 Note for Guidance on Quality of Water for Pharmaceutical Use

Sr. No	Sterile Medicine product	Minimum Acceptable Quality of Water
1	Oral Preparation	Purified Water Purified
2	Nebuliser Solutions	Purified*
3	Cutaneous Preparations	Purified Water **

Contd....

Sr. No	Sterile Medicine product	Minimum Acceptable Quality of Water
4	Nasal/Ear Preparations	Purified Water
5	Rectal/Vaginal Preparation	Purified Water
*	In certain disease states eg: cystic fibrosis, medicinal products administered by nebulisation are required to be sterile and non-Pyrogenic. In such cases WFI or sterilized Highly Purified water should be used	
**	For some products such as veterinary teat dips it may be acceptable to use potable water where justified and authorized taking account of the variability in chemical composition and microbiological quality.	

21.11 Type of Water is used in the Manufacturer of Active Pharmaceutical Ingredients (APIs) as per EMEA / CVMP / 115 / 01 Note for Guidance on Quality of Water for Pharmaceutical Use

Sr. No	Type of Manufacture	Product requirement	Minimum Acceptable Quality of Water
1	Synthesis of all intermediates of APIs prior to final isolation and purification	No requirement for sterility or apyrogenicity in API or the pharmaceutical product in which it will be used.	Potable Water *
2	Fermentation media	No requirement for sterility or apyrogenicity in API or the pharmaceutical product in which it will be used.	Potable Water *
3	Extraction of herbals	No requirement for sterility or apyrogenicity in API or the pharmaceutical product in which it will be used.	Potable Water **
4	Final isolation and purification	No requirement for sterility or apyrogenicity in API or the pharmaceutical product in which it will be used.	Potable Water *
5	Final isolation and purification	API is not sterile ,but is intended for use in a sterile, non- parenteral	Purified Water
6	Final isolation and purification	API is sterile and not intended for parenteral	Purified Water

Contd....

Sr. No	Type of Manufacture	Product requirement	Minimum Acceptable Quality of Water
7	Final isolation and purification	API is not sterile, but is intended for use in a sterile parenteral product.	Purified Water with an Endotoxin limit of 0.25 EU/ml and control of specific organisms.
8	Final isolation and purification	API is sterile and apyrogenic	Purified Water
*	Purified Water should be used where there are technical requirements for greater purity.		
**	The Applicant need to demonstrate that potential variations in the water quality, particularly with respect to mineral composition, would not influence the composition of the extract.		

21.12 Type of Water is used for Cleaning/Rrinsing of Equipment, Containers and Closure as per EMEA / CVMP / 115 / 01 Note for Guidance on Quality of Water for Pharmaceutical Use

Sr. No	Cleaning/Rinsing of equipment, Container, Closures	Product requirement	Minimum Acceptable Quality of Water
1	Initial Rise	Intermediate and API	Potable Water
2	Final Rinse	API	Use same quality of Water as used in the API manufacturer
3	Initial rinse including CIP* of equipment, containers and closure, if applicable	Pharmaceutical products non sterile	Potable Water
4	Final rinse including CIP* of equipment, containers and closure, if applicable	Pharmaceutical products non sterile	Purified Water or use same quality of water as used in manufacture of medicinal product ,if higher quality than Purified Water
5	Initial rinse** including CIP* of equipment, containers and closure, if applicable	Sterile Products	Purified Water

Contd....

Sr. No	Cleaning/Rinsing of equipment, Container, Closures	Product requirement	Minimum Acceptable Quality of Water
6	Final rinse*** including CIP* of equipment, containers and closure, if applicable	Sterile non-parenteral products	Purified Water or use same quality of water as used in manufacture of medicinal product ,if higher quality than Purified Water
7	Final rinse*** including CIP* of equipment, containers and closure, if applicable	Sterile parenteral products	Water for Injection****
*	CIP =Clean In Place		
**	Some containers, e.g. plastic containers for eye drops may not need an initial rinse, this may be counter-productive since particulates counts could be increased as a result n some cases e.g.: Blow-fill-seal processes rinsing cannot be applied		
***	If equipment is dried after rinsing with % alcohol, the alcohol should be diluted in water of the same quality as the water used for final rinse		
****	Where a subsequent depyrogenisation step is employed the use of Highly Purified Water may be acceptable subjected to suitable justification and validation data		

21.13 Potable Water as per Reference ISPE Baseline Guide, Volume-4 Water and Steam System, WHO TRS 929 WHO TRS 937

A. Construction Requirement of Underground and Overage Storage Tank:

- Raw water storage tank (Underground storage tank and overage tank) shall be made of Reinforced cement and epoxy lining.
- High-density polyethylene pipe work is preferred for underground systems. Copper, PVC, CPVC (chlorinated polyvinyl chloride) , PEX pipe , Kitec pipe (aluminum tube which is laminated to plastic layers on the inside and the outside of the pipe.) or Galvanized Steel is preferred for above ground pipe.
- Air break shall be available to the pipe work.
- Storage tank must be closed with vents, Breathing filters and overflows to protect the ingress of insects, birds and vermin.

- Underground storage shall also consist of level sensor, dosing, pump system and prefilteration system.
- Distribution of water can be done by gravity feed or by means of pump system.

B. Control of Microbial Load in Potable Water:

- Sodium hypochlorite is used as chlorinating agent to reduce microbial growth.
- Normally 2-5 ppm concentration of sodium hypochlorite is used for dosing.
- Dosing is done by dosing unit which depends on the pH, concentration and residence time.

C. Dechlorination of Feed Water:

- Dechlorination is done by dosing Sodium Metabisulphite to remove excess chlorine or ozone from raw water to protect RO membrane.
- Procedure for preparation method for Sodium Metabisulphite shall be available.
- Records shall be available for the Sodium Metabisulphite.
- 0.5 mg/L free chlorine level shall be maintain in water throughout the distribution.

D. Procedure and Limit of Hardness:

- Hardness is measured at sampling points after the softener, with off-line test kits that use chemical reagents (colorimeter) to get a semi-quantitative response.
- If online hardness measurement system is used, it should be qualified and calibrated.

E. Procedure and limit of Oxidation Reduction Potential (ORP):

- ORP should be used before RO system to ensure the elimination of harmful oxidizing substance prior to contact with RO membranes.
- Measurement shall be on-line or off line.
- If ORP instrument is used, it should be qualified and calibrated.

- Check the availability of dumping valve after ORP meter.

F. Procedure and Limit of Silt Density Indicator:

- Slit density is checked by Nephalometers.
- Installed before sand filter.
- Tests shall be conducted off line or line.
- The maximum allowable NTU for reverse osmosis (RO) is 5.

G. Procedure for Microbial-Retentive Filters in Potable Water Line:

- Procedure and records for replacement of the Microbial-Retentive filter shall be available.
- Usage time for microbial filters shall be available.
- Pressure gauge if available shall be calibrated.

H. Potable Water Sampling and Testing:

- Check the sampling plan and sampling procedure.
- Raw water shall routinely monitor for Parameters concerning toxic substances, radioactive substance and Pesticide residue.
- Microbiological: Coliform parameter. Total Viable count 500 cfu/1ml.

21.14 Purified Water and WFI System as per ISPE Baseline Guide, Volume 4 Water and Steam System, WHO TRS 929 WHO TRS 937

A. Design Requirement for Distribution of Purified Water and WFI System:

- Isometric Diagram with number of loop and joint numbering, Pipelines: MOCSS-316L,Slope of pipelines: 1 : 100 ,Smooth internal finish: Roughness of not greater than 0.8 micrometer (Ra), Pump, Design of flanges, sampling valve or unions : Sanitary type, Dead legs in the pipe work : NMT 1.5, Material certificates for pipes and fittings, FDA Food Grade certificates for gaskets, Compatibility and Prevention of leaching, Jointing : Easily joint without leakage and Passivation/ Passivation protocol : Citric Acid, 70% Nitric Acid.

B. Storage Tank Design Requirement for Purified Water / WFI System:

- Capacity and MOC : SS-316L ,Flow direct valve or Back divert valve ,Rupture disc, Spray ball ,Sanitary valve, Compound gauge, Pressure gauge, Safety valve, Vent filter : Hydrophobic and Jacket Storage tank if applicable.

C. Welding Document Requirement during Design Qualification:

- Isometric drawings with weld numbers, Welded seam documentation (machine protocols), Welder approval test certificate, Endoscopic photos, Boroscopic documents and Analytical certificate of inert gas : Argon gas

D. Flow Velocity of Purified Water and WFI in Distribution Loop:

- A distribution system is designed to operate with nominal flow velocities of 2 to 3 feet per second or higher.

E. Conductivity Sensor:

- Online conductivity sensor should be installed in distribution line and Conductivity meter shall be qualified and calibrated at regular frequency.

F. Pressure and Compound Gauge available in Purified Water and WFI System:

- Positive pressure shall be maintained with respect to surrounding at all times of operation.
- Pressure gauge shall calibrated at defined frequency and record shall be maintained.
- Compound gauge shall be always be at "zero' and shall be calibrated at defined frequency and records of calibration shall be maintained.

G. Sampling Procedure is for Purified and Water for Injection as per USP Chapter <1231>:

- Sampling plan and procedure shall be available.
- Sample should be sampled by trained person in accordance with sampling plan.

- Sample shall be collected in same scenario as used in manufacturing facility. E.g If water is collected through the silicon pipe then same shall be collected from silica pipe for analysis.
- Sample should be test as soon as possible after collection. If it is not possible to test the sample within about 2 hrs of collection, the sample should held at refrigerator temperatures(2°-8° C) for a maximum of about 12 hours to maintain the microbial attributes until analysis. In situation where even this is not possible (such as when using off -site contract laboratories), testing of these refrigerated samples should be performed within 48 hours after sample collection.
- In delay testing scenario, the recovered microbiological levels may not be the same as would have been recovered had the testing been performed shortly after sample collection. Therefore, studies should be performed to deter mine the existence and acceptability of potential microbial enumeration aberrations caused by protracted testing delays.

H. Alert and Action Levels defined for Purified and Water for Injection:

- Alert and Action levels shall be derived from an evaluation of historic monitoring data called as trend analysis.
- In new systems where there is very limited or no historic data available, alert and action limit shall be based on equipment design capabilities, but below the process and product specification where water is used.
- An action level shall not be established at a level equivalent to the specification.

I. Continuous System Monitoring of Purified Water and Water for Injection System:

- Online Monitoring such as flow, pressure, temperature, conductivity and total organic carbon.
- Samples from points of use shall be taken in a similar manner replicating to that adopted the water during actual usage.

- Tests shall be carried as per Approved Specification.
- Monitoring data shall be subject to trend analysis.
- Systems shall be maintained in accordance with a controlled documented maintenance programme.

J. **System Reviews of Purified Water and Water for Injection System:**

- At Regular interval system review shall be conducted. And an Annual Water System Report shall be prepared to check the performance of system.

21.15 Planned Preventive Maintenance Programme

A. **Potable/Purified/WFI/Pure Steam:**

- Each and every equipment and instrument which are used in water system shall have approved calibration and planned preventive maintenance procedure.
- Planned Preventive Maintenance schedule shall be checked during audit.
- Calibration records of the instrument and equipment shall be checked with schedule and limit. E.g.: Compound guage, pressure gauge etc.

B. **Alarm Management for Purified/WFI/Pure Steam:**

- Alarm management system shall be available and each and every alarm notification shall be timely investigation and recorded.
- Trend analysis for alarm generated shall be performed.

C. **RO Membrane Maintenance:**

- Check the procedure and records for the cleaning, sanitization and replacement of RO membrane.
- RO units usually need periodic cleaning and sanitization (Normally done once in six month or manufacturer's recommendation).
- RO membrane shall be sanitized with chemical agents or material recommended by the supplier.
- Specially constructed membranes are available for hot water sanitization at 60°C to 80°C.

- Anti-scalent chemicals are used to minimize scaling of RO membrane. Procedure for preparation and records shall be checked.

D. **Ion Exchange Membrane Maintenance:**

- Check the procedure and for preparation methods for regenerating cataon and anion beads.
- Check the records for the replacement of Ion exchange membrane

E. **Continuous Electro Deionization (CEDI) or Electron De-ionization (EDI) Maintenance:**

- Check the procedure and record for preparation of sanitizing agent and frequency of sanitization.
- CBDI chemically sanitized by peracetic acid, sodium percarbonate, sodium hydroxide or hydrogen peroxide.
- Hot water sanitization is normally used for specific CEDI module.

F. **Total Organic Carbon (TOC):**

- Check the procedure and record for calibration of TOC meter.
- Calibration of TOC at least six monthly or replacement of UV lamp.
- System suitability is carried out by using water Benzoquione solution or Sucrose. The system is suitable if the response efficiency is not less than 85% and not more than 115% of the theoretical.
- TOC should not be more than 500ppb.

G. **Sanitization for Purified and Water for Injection System:**

- Sanitization shall be done by Hot water (NLT 80°C)/Pure Steam and Ozone (0.1ppm).
- Storage tank, distribution loop and inline equipment shall be sanitized according to the validated parameter and approved SOP. Sanitization records shall be checked.
- Sanitization parameter shall be checked with validated parameter.
- Pump replacement record shall be available.

- Sanitization of system shall be done when the equipment are removed for the calibration.

H. Ultra Violet lamp:

- Lamp replacement records shall be available.
- Intensity of lamp shall be define in the SOP.

I. Cleaning:

a. Cleaning Frequency of Underground and Overage Storage Tank:

- Procedure and frequency for cleaning of underground and overage shall be available.
- Underground and Overage storage tank shall cleaned periodically and record shall be maintained.

b. Preventive maintenance Multigrade Filter Used for Filtration of Potable Water:

- Procedure and frequency for cleaning of Multigrade shall be available.
- Regular back wash system shall be available. A back wash of water depends on the quality of feed water.
- Sand or multimedia filtrates are regenerated using nitric acid periodically (Once in year or Manufacturer recommendation).
- Records for preventive maintenance shall be available which includes valve functioning and checking of back wash.

21.16 Definition

- **Back Wash:** The process of flowing water in the opposite direction from normal service flow.
- **Elecropolishing:** Controlled electro chemical process utilizing acid electrolyte, DC current, anode and cathode to smooth the surface by removal of metal.
- **Hardness:** A concentration of calcium and magnesium salts in water.
- **Membrane:** A barrier, which permits the passage only of particles up to a certain size or specific nature.

- **Ozone:** Ozone is a very strong gaseous oxidizing agent. It is used to kill bacteria.
- **Passivations:** Removal of exogeneous iron or iron compounds from the surface of a stainless steel by means of chemical dissolution.
- **Sanitary Design:** A system of design that meets standards, specification, code , regulatory and industrial guideline and acceptable engineering design methods to reach a degree of sanitation by food, pharmaceutical and cosmetics processing.
- **Softening:** Removal of hardness (calcium and magnesium) from water.

CHAPTER 22

Pharmaceutical Heating, Ventilation and Air Conditionings (HVAC) and Regulatory Expectations

Introduction

HVAC system is one of the utility system that provides right environmental condition of temperature, humidity and pressure differential for pharmaceutical product. The HVAC system should be appropriately designed, installed and maintained to ensure protection of product, personnel and the environment. Design criteria shall be preferably based on a shell-like building layout to enhance containment and protection from external contaminants.

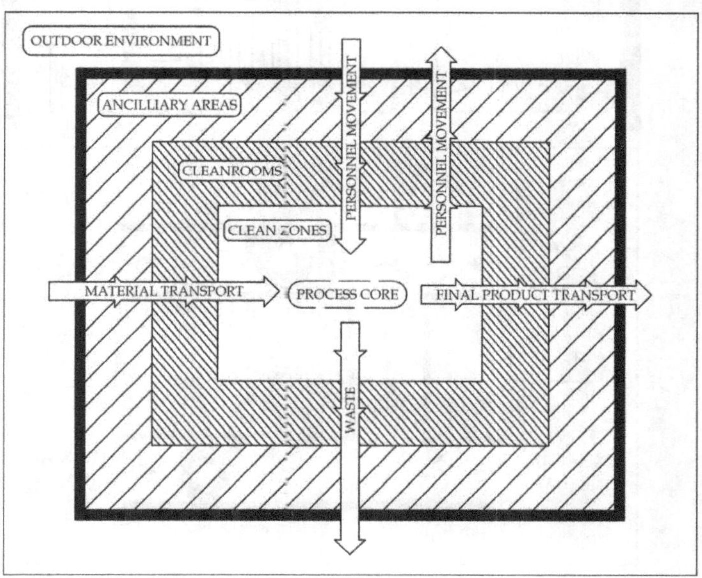

22.1 Qualification

A. Designed Qualification:

- Below basic criteria shall be considered in designed qualification; but not limited to: Outside air conditions, building finishes and structure, Air filtration, air change rate or flushing rate, Room pressure, Location of air terminals and directional airflow, Temperature and relative humidity, Material flow and personnel flow, Equipment movement, Process being carried out (open or closed system), Occupancy, Type of product, Cleaning standard operating procedures (SOPs) and gowning procedures. And Lux intensity and sound
- **Typical HVAC System and its components are described below:**

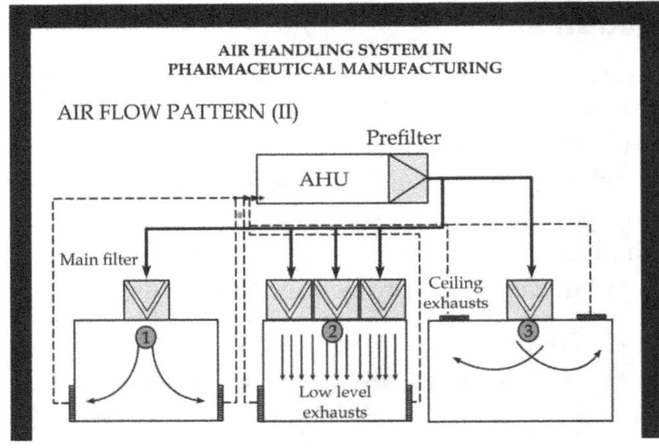

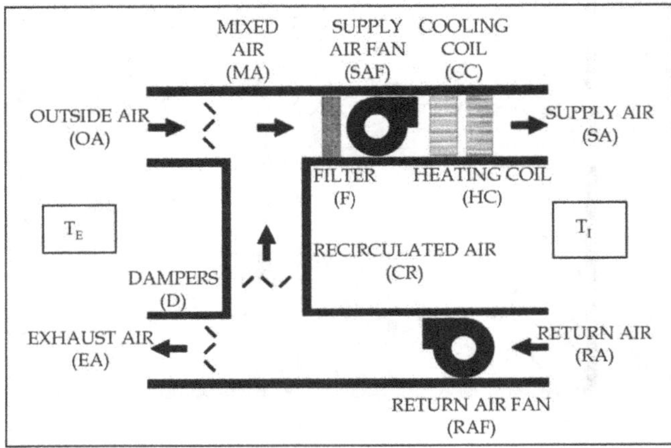

Air handling unit design

(i) **Mixing Chamber:** The mixing chamber is the location in which the supply air and the return air are mixed, so that the supply air is relatively uniform in temperature.

(ii) **Blower:** Blower fans move air, and their speed may be used to control the airflow rate.

(iii) **Heating and Cooling Units:** These units heat and cool the air. In addition, the cooling unit also removes some excess humidity from the supply air through condensation.

(iv) **Dehumidifier:** Dehumidification (moisture removal) is done by means of either refrigerated dehumidifiers or chemical dehumidifiers by using a non-shedding desiccant, such as silica gel or lithium chloride and should not support microbial growth

(v) **Humidifier:** Humidifiers inject water vapor (pure or clean steam) into the supply air stream to increase humidity condition by air. There are different type of humidifier such as direct steam injection humidifier, heated pan humidifier and Wet element humidifier. Drained system shall be available to drain the condensate. Final air filters shall not be installed immediately downstream of humidifiers

(vi) **Ducting:** Ducts are available for supply, return and exhaust of air and are made up of Galvanic steel.

(vii) **Insulation:** Insulation on the exterior surface of Duct work is done for thermal efficiency and to prevent condensation.

(viii) **Damper:** Dampers are used for control air flow by open closed mechanism.

(ix) **Diffusers:** A mixing or displacement system is created by the type and location of supply diffusers. Perforated plate diffuser and Swirl diffuser are recommended in clean area.

(x) **Dust Collector:** Dust collectors are used for removing dust from dust extractor systems.

Type of Dust Collector:

a. **Reverse Pulse Dust Collectors:** Equipped with cartridge filters containing a compressed air lance, and operate continuously without interrupting the airflow.

b. **Mechanical Shaker Dust Collectors:** Continuous airflow is required as fan is switched off when the mechanical shaker is activated which can disrupt the pressure cascade.

(xi) **Scrubbers:** Fumes should be removed by means of wet scrubbers or dry chemical scrubbers (deep-bed scrubbers).

a. Wet scrubbers for fume removal normally require the addition of various chemicals to the water to increase the adsorption efficiency.

b. Deep-bed scrubbers should be designed with activated carbon filters or granular chemical adsorption media. The chemical media for deep-bed scrubbers should be specific to the effluent being treated.

c. The dust-slurry should be removed by a suitable drainage system.

d. Selection of media/filter depends on type and volume of the effluent being treated. Dust Point is about 100 mm of the point of exhaust designed velocity with 15-20 m/s. The exhaust air quality should be determined to see whether the filtration efficiency is adequate with all types of dust collectors and wet scrubbers. Power failure systems shall be available to prevent backflow of residues from the ductwork. Central dust extraction systems shall be interlocked.

(xii) **Building Management System (BMS):** Sophisticated computer-based data monitoring systems may be installed. An automated monitoring system should be capable of indicating any out-of-specification condition without delay by means of an alarm or similar system.

(xiii) Pressure Differential: Room pressurization from areas of highest cleanliness to area of low cleanliness. Doors shall open in tc the high pressure side or shall be provide with self-closers. Air lock prevents DP between air classes from dropping to zero when doors are opened between classes. Pressure difference should be monitored between room to room or room to common reference point. The limits for the pressure differential between adjacent areas shall be such that there is no risk of overlap in the acceptable operating range. Different types of air locks are as follows:

a. **Cascade airlock:** High pressure on one side of the airlock and low pressure on the other side.

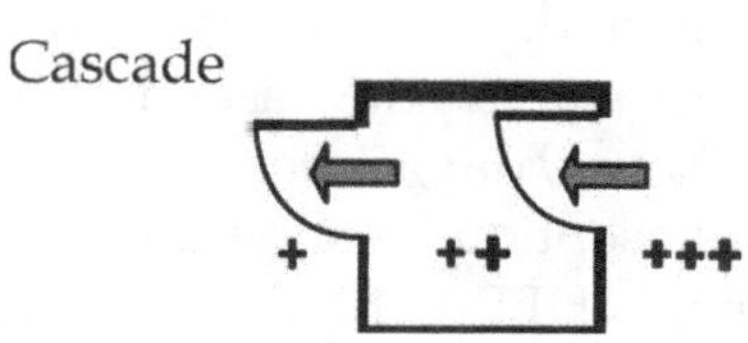

b. **Sink airlock:** Low pressure inside the airlock and high pressure on both outer sides.

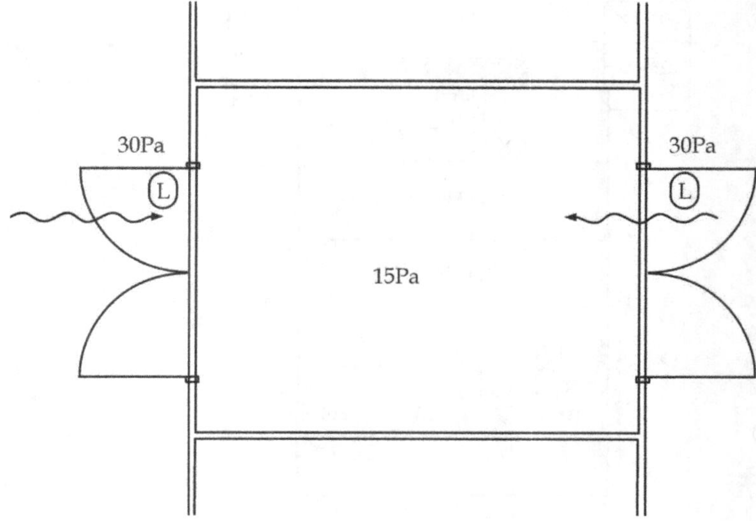

c. **Bubble airlock:** High pressure inside the airlock and low pressure on both outer sides.

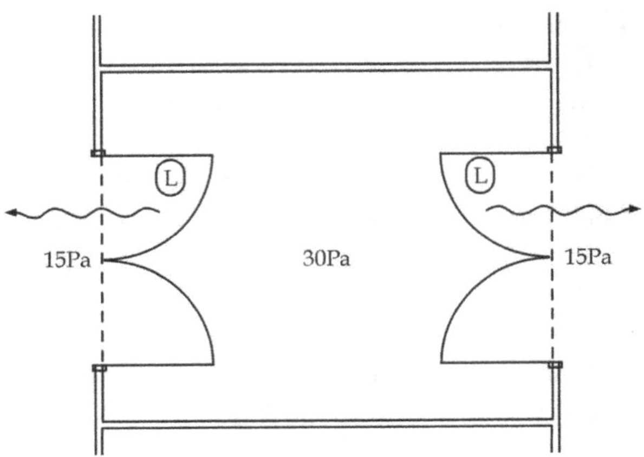

I. Aseptic Dosage Form Facility:

AHUs shall be located in cleaned environment and supply air should be prefiltered. A dedicated air handling system is recommended to serve the aseptic areas and to remain operational (24 hours/day, 7 days/week) to maintain pressure control. Air to an aseptic area should be supplied through ceiling mounted terminal HEPA filters (H13/H14). These terminal HEPA filters become part of the aseptic boundary and protect the room from outside contamination.

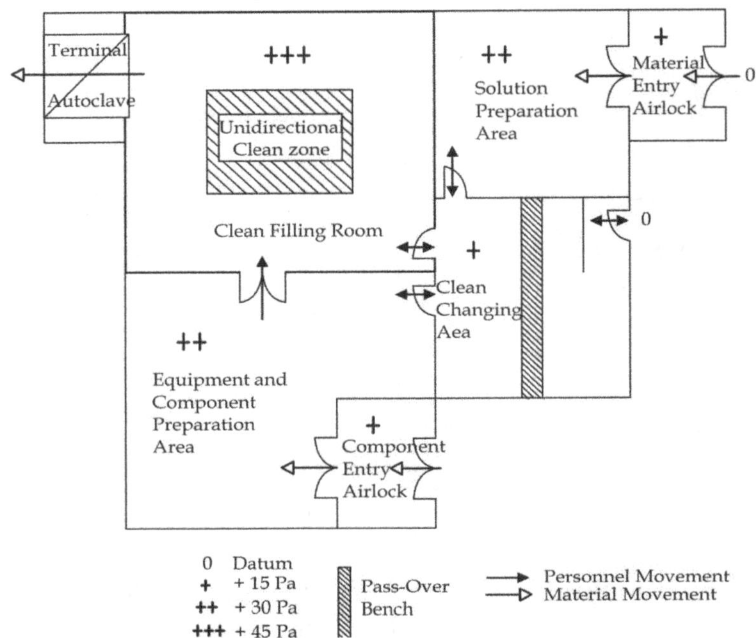

II. Check Points for Design Qualification for Aseptic and Biologics area:

(i) **Air handling system is recommended in Aseptic area** (Reference: ISPE Good Practice and Guide for HVAC) : A dedicated air handling system is recommended to serve only the aseptic areas and to remain operational to maintain pressure control when other building systems are shut down during unoccupied periods.

(ii) **HVAC system is operated in aseptic classified area:** HVAC systems for classified spaces should operate 24 hours/day, 7 days/week.

(iii) **Layout are considered in design of HVAC system (Non-Potent and Potent: Aseptic / Solid / Semi Solids / Liquids / Final API facility):** (Reference: WHOTRS 961, Annex-5 and 937 and ISPE- HVAC): Man Material entry layout, Area Classification layout, Pressure difference layout and List of area for temperature and Humidity.

(iv) **Type of HAVAC system is used in facility (Non-Potent and Potent: Aseptic / Solid / Semi Solids / Liquids / Final API facility):** (Reference: WHOTRS 961, Annex-5 and 937 and ISPE- HVAC): Full fresh air system or recirculation air system. Where Solvents are handled, 100% exhaust system is recommended.

(v) **Final filtration of Aseptic area:** Air to an aseptic area should be supplied through ceiling mounted terminal HEPA filters (H13/H14).

a. **Pre-filters:** EU-10 & EU-9 or EU-7 or EU-6or EU-4

b. **Plenum Filtration**: HEPA: H-13 **(Efficacy:** 99.95)

c. **Terminal Filter:** HEPA: H-14 (Efficacy: 99.995)

(vi) **The room cascade is designed in aseptic area** (Reference: WHOTRS 961, Annex-5 and 937 and ISPE- HVAC): Room pressurization is designed to cascade from area of highest cleanliness to areas of lower cleanliness.

(vii) **The return air opening in aseptic area** (Reference: ISPE- HVAC): The return air openings in the aseptic area should be located near the floor, preferably on at least two walls and along the long dimensions of a room to ensure maximum uniformity of airflow. Equipment and furniture (Like Tools, Dustbin) should not block return openings.

(viii) **Differential pressure between different grades in aseptic area?** (Reference: ISPE- HVAC): The design DP measured between different grade rooms, inclusive of airlocks, should be held between 10Pa to 15Pa with the door in their closed position. The room with exposed product is to be maintained most positive; while anterooms leading to this room are to be maintained successively less positive .Where rooms are of the same cleanliness class, a more critical room may be the same pressure, but usually slightly higher. The aseptic area should be designed for a positive pressure with all doors closed in relative to less clean adjacent areas outside the controlled space. A control range should be established for each room pressure level, such that the pressure can float within the range and continue to satisfy the specified differentials. Gowning areas are treated as airlocks with supply and return air, and are maintained at a negative pressure relative to the controlled aseptic area and at a positive pressure relative to the outside and uncontrolled spaces. Where potent product is open-filled and may become airborne, a high-pressure containment airlock that meets the filling room air grade may have pressure higher than the aseptic filling room. DPs are measured across airlocks.

(ix) **The interlock system of AHU Non-Potent and Potent: Aseptic /Solid/Semi Solids/Liquids/ Final API facility shall work:** There shall be procedure for the sequence of AHU ON-OFF system. Higher classified area /pressure area AHU shall be started first followed by less classified area /pressure area, where as during trip or shut down of AHU Lower classified area /pressure area shall be shut down first followed by Higher classified area /pressure area.

(x) **Gowning and de-gowning area in aseptic area?** (Reference: ISPE- HVAC).Gowning areas should be supplied with HEPA filtered air and maintained at a negative pressure relative to controlled aseptic area and at a positive pressure relative to the uncontrolled spaces.

The gowning area should be separated from the Grade 7 (EU Grade B) aseptic room by a high pressure Grade 7 (Grade B) airlock. The de-gowning area should be separated from the aseptic filling room by a low-pressure airlock. The de-gowning room shall be maintained negative relative to adjacent spaces on the uncontrolled side.

(xi) **Types of Grade are used in Aseptic area** (Reference: Eudralex Annex-1): For the manufacture of sterile medicinal products 4 grades can be distinguished.

- **Grade A:** The local zone for high risk operations, e.g. filling zone, stopper bowls, open ampoules and vials, making aseptic connections. Laminar air flow systems should provide a homogeneous air speed in a range of 0.36 - 0.54 m/s at the working position in open clean room applications. A uni-directional air flow and lower velocities may be used in closed isolators and glove boxes.
- **Grade B:** For aseptic preparation and filling, this is the background environment for the grade A zone.
- **Grade C and D:** Clean areas for carrying out less critical stages in the manufacture of sterile products.

(xii) **Direction of the Doors opening in the processing area (Non-Potent and Potent: Aseptic /Solid/Semi Solids/Liquids/ Final API facility)?** (Reference: WHOTRS 961,Annex-5 and 937 and ISPE- HVAC):Doors should open to the high pressure side, so that room pressure assists in holding the door closed and in addition be provided with self closers.

(xiii) **Clean room requirements for permitted particles** (Reference: Eudralex Annex-1): Following are the requirements for Clean room and clean air device classification:

Table 22.1: Maximum permitted number of particles

Maximum permitted number of particles per m³ equal to or greater than the tabulated size				
Grade	At rest (b)		In Operation (a)	
	0.5µm	5µm	0.5µm	5µm
A	35,20	20	35,00	20
B	35,200	29	3,52000	290
C	3,52000	2900	35,20,000	2900
D	35,20,000	29000	Not defined (c)	Not defined (c)
For classification purposes in Grade A zones, a minimum sample volume of 1m³ should be taken per sample location. For Grade A the airborne particle classification is ISO 4.8 dictated by the limit for particles ≥5.0 µm. For Grade B (at rest) the airborne particle classification is ISO 5 for both considered particle sizes. For Grade C (at rest & in operation) the airborne particle classification is ISO 7 and ISO 8 respectively. For Grade D (at rest) the airborne particle classification is ISO 8. For classification purposes EN/ISO 14644-1 methodology defines both the minimum number of sample locations and the sample size based on the class limit of the largest considered particle size and the method of evaluation of the data collected.				
b: The requirement and limit for the area shall depend on the nature of the operation carried out.				
c: Type of operations to be carried out in the various grades are given in Table II and Table III as under.				

(xiv) Sterile dosage preparation, filtration and filling of product are done(Reference: Eudralex Annex-1)**:** Types of Operations to be Carried Out in The Various area:

Grade For Aseptic Preparations	**Types of operations for aseptic preparations**	**Types of operations for terminally sterilized products**
A	Aseptic preparation and filling	Aseptic preparation and filling, when unusually at risk
B	Background room conditions for activities requiring Grade A	-
C	Preparation of solution to be filtered	Preparation of solutions, when unusually at risk. Filling of products
D	Handling of components after washing	Moulding, blowing (pre-forming) operations of plastic containers, preparations of solutions and components for subsequent filling.

(xv) The recommended limits for Microbiological Monitoring of clean area operation (Reference: Eudralex Annex-1) Table II: limits for Microbiological Monitoring of Clean areas in operation:

Recommended limits for Microbiological Monitoring of Clean areas in operation:				
Grade	Air sample CFU /m³	Settle plates (dia. 90mm.) CFU/2 hrs.	Contact plates (dia.55mm) CFU per plate	Glove points (five fingers) CFU per glove
A	< 1	< 1	< 1	< 1
B	10	5	5	5
C	100	50	25	--
D	200	100	50	--
a) These are average values. b) Individual settle plates may be exposed for less than 4 hours.				

(xvi) The frequencies for Environmental monitoring in clean area operation? (Reference: Eudralex Annex-1): Table III: limits for Environment Monitoring of Clean areas in operation.

Environmental Monitoring	
Air pressure differentials	Daily
Temperature and humidity	Daily
Microbiological monitoring	Daily in aseptic areas and at decreased frequency in other areas
The above frequencies of monitoring shall be changed as per the requirements and load in individual cases	
Note: Appropriate alert and action limits should be set for the results of particulate and microbiological monitoring. If these limits are exceeded operating procedures should prescribe corrective action	

(xvii) Air changes classifications for classified area in operation condition (Non-Potent and Potent: Aseptic /Solid/Semi Solids/Liquids/ Final API facility) (Reference: ISPE HVAC): Table IV: Air changes classification in operation:

Class of clean room	**Air change rate per hour (ISPE)**
Unclassified area	**No minimum Air changes are defined**
ISO 8	20
ISO 7	40
ISO 6	40
≤ ISO 5	60

(xviii) **The dust extraction system designed in the processing area (Non-Potent and Potent: Aseptic /Solid/Semi Solids/Liquids/ Final API facility** (Reference: WHOTRS 961, Annex-5 and ISPE- HVAC): Central dust extraction systems should be interlocked with the appropriate air-handling systems, to ensure that they operate simultaneously. Air should not flow through the dust extraction ducting or return air ducting from the room with the higher pressure to the room with the lower pressure. Systems should be designed to prevent dust flowing back in the opposite direction in the event of component failure or airflow failure.

(xix) **The velocity air in the dust collector (Non-Potent and Potent: Aseptic /Solid/Semi Solids/Liquids/ Final API facility)** Reference: WHOTRS 961, Annex-5 and 937): The required transfer velocity should be determined: it is dependent on the density of the dust (the denser the dust, the higher the transfer velocity should be, e.g. 15–20 m/s).

(xx) **The efficacy test of dust collector (Non-Potent and Potent: Aseptic /Solid/Semi Solids/Liquids/ Final API facility)?** (Reference: WHOTRS 961, Annex-5 and ISPE-HVAC):The exhaust air quality should be determined to see whether the filtration efficiency is adequate with all types of dust collectors and wet scrubbers.

(xxi) **Damper that closes, preventing air leaving system (Non-Potent and Potent: Aseptic/Solid/Semi Solids/Liquids/ Final API facility** (Reference: WHOTRS 961, Annex-5 and ISPE- HVAC): Gravity damper shall be present in dust collector to prevent cross contamination by air.

(xxii) **The failure of dust collector will affect the pressure difference in the area (Non-Potent and Potent: Aseptic /Solid/Semi Solids/Liquids/ Final API facility)** (Reference: WHOTRS 961, Annex-5 and ISPE- HVAC): Dust collector should start with HVAC system. Pressure difference with respect to area and dust collector shall be qualified during qualification. Central dust extraction systems shall be interlocked.

(xxiii) **The check points for damper (Non-Potent and Potent: Aseptic /Solid/Semi Solids/Liquids/ Final API facility):** Supply air damper, Return air damper and Exhaust air damper shall be available in the system with interlock or position mark at the validated parameter.

(xxiv) **The final filtration of dust collector before release in the environment (Non-Potent and Potent: Aseptic /Solid/Semi Solids/Liquids/ Final API facility)?** (Reference: WHOTRS 961, Annex-5): Powders which are not highly potent: Filters classification of F9 (EU9) according to EN779 filter standards. For the harmful substances such as penicillin, hormones, toxic powders and enzymes. The final filters should be HEPA filters with at least an H12 classification according to EN1822 filter standards. For hazardous material, two banks of HEPA filters in series or "bag-in-bag-out" filter, to provide additional protection should the first filter fail. All filter banks should be provided with pressure differential indication gauges to indicate the filter dust loading and remaining life span of the filters.

(xxv) **Tests are to be performed during Qualification and Periodic Verification of HVAC (Non-Potent and Potent: Aseptic /Solid/Semi Solids/Liquids/ Final API facility):** (Reference: WHOTRS 961,Annex-5,ISO14644, ISPE- HVAC): Room Temperature distribution study for determination of Hot and cold point, Temperature and relative humidity; supply air quantities for all diffusers; return air or exhaust air quantities; room air change rates; room pressures (pressure differentials); room airflow patterns; unidirectional flow velocities and containment system velocities; HEPA filter penetration tests; room particle counts; room clean-up rates; microbiological air and surface counts where appropriate; Warning/alarm systems where applicable. Recommended Tests are specified in below table:

Test Parameter	Objective	Maximum time interval	Test procedure* and key aspects
Schedule of tests to demonstrate continuing compliance:			
Particle count test ISO 14644-1,Annex B	Particle counter. Readings and positions	6 months or 12 months depending on Class	Verifies cleanliness
Measure pressure difference ISO 14644-3 Annex B4	Absence of cross-contamination	12 months	Air pressure difference
Measure supply and return air, calculate air change rate	Verify air change rates	12 months	Airflow volume
Velocity measurement ISO 14644-3 Annex B4	Verify unidirectional airflow and or containment condition	12 months	Airflow velocity
Recommended optional strategic tests /Optional Test:			
Installed filter leakage ISO 14644-3 Annex B6	24 months	Verify filter integrity	Filter leakage
Air flow Visualization ISO 14644-3 Annex B7	24 months	Verify required airflow patterns	Airflow visualization
Recovery ISO 14644-3Annex B13	24 months	Verify clean-up time	Recovery (time)
Containment leakage ISO 14644-3Annex B4	24 months	Verify absence of cross-contamination	Containment leakage
*Test procedure as per ISO 14644			

III. Design Criteria for Solid / Semi Solids / Liquids / Final API:

- Solid / Semi Solid / Liquid / Final API dosage form processing room shall be capable of meeting Grade D (ISO 8) at rest for monitoring of particles. Clean air lock (pressure bubble or pressure sink) into the highest contamination area are strongly recommended. Where solvents are used, this configuration is recommended to prevent migration of flammable vapors to the building. Monitoring and alarm system of direction of air flow (through DP, velocity sensor, air balance, flow tracking) to surrounding rooms is required. For low RH product dehumidifier can be used. Return or exhaust air grills may be equipped with easily removable dust stop filters.

- Recirculation systems with adequate filtration may be applied in multi-product areas where solvents are present. Multi product manufacturing may required dual HEPA filtration (one supply and one return) for recirculation systems. Multi product manufacturing typically uses pressure bubble or pressure sink airlocks to avoid contamination of the common corridor. Single product or multi product campaign facilities may employ a pressurized (bubble) common corridor and air lock to the process area. A typical HVAC Flow for Oral Solid Dosage form is brief below:

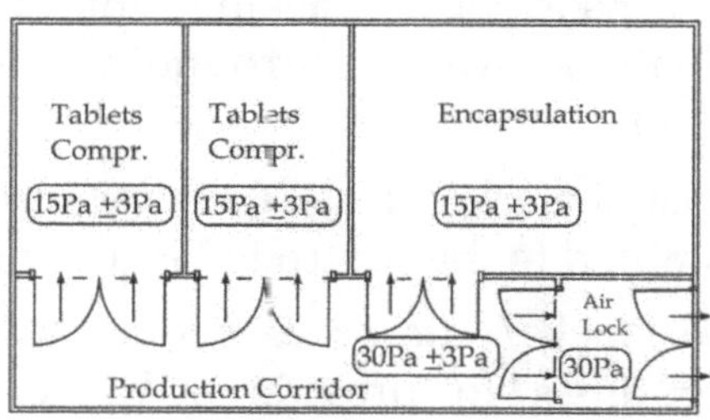

Design Condition

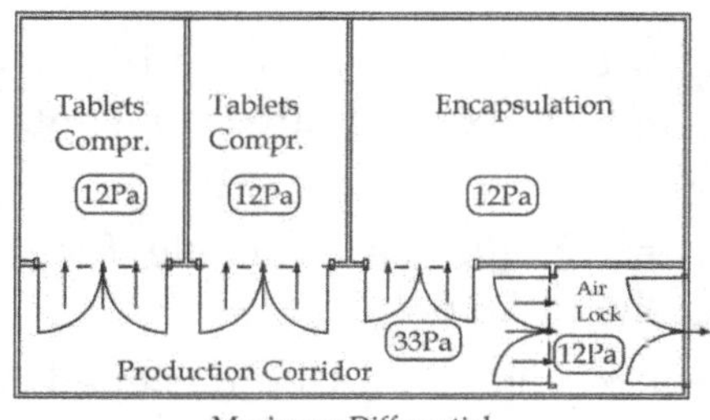

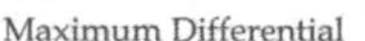
Maximum Differential

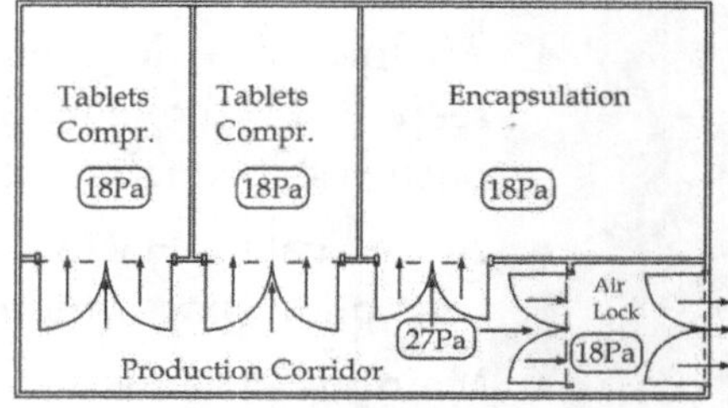

Maximum Differential

IV. Design Criteria for Potent Solid / Semi Solids / Liquids / Final API Form:

- Potent Drug (Hormone / Cytotoxics) facilities should be separate, dedicated facilities and should not form part of any other non-hormone facility. They may be in the same building as another facility but should be separated by a physical barrier and have separate entrances, staff facilities, air-handling systems, etc. The facility should be maintained at a negative air pressure to the environment.

- Processing room in the Solid / Semi Solids / Liquids / Final API form shall be capable of meeting Grade D (ISO 8) at rest for monitoring of particles. Minimum filtration H13/14 in the supply if a 100% once through system.
- Closed containment is the primary means of airborne contamination control for this class of material. If processes are proven closed, recirculated air should include HEPA filtration. If the process is not proven closed, once-through air or double HEPA filtration should be considered.
- Exhaust should be provided at locations were containment is opened for introduction or removal of materials or in conjunction with other technologies, as required.
- Isolation via active control of direction of airflow (using DP, velocity sensor, flow tracking) into the area of highest contamination from surrounding areas is strongly maintained.
- Audio-visual alert on loss of airflow or containment should be transmitted to the controlled space for personnel safety.
- Room air locks/anterooms should available for powder handling areas to provide a barrier that maintains a positive airflow differential with respect to the corridor and the processing room.
- Airflow into de-gowning areas should be negative with respect to the corridor and processing area to contain particles shed from clothing.
- A dedicated HVAC system should be available for the controlled space where product is exposed.
- Main air systems for these rooms should be designed for 100% exhaust, once-through supply. However, when processes are enclosed, air recirculation with HEPA filtration should be justified.

- Recirculation of air from the controlled space into other areas and Recirculation of exhaust from equipment back to the room should not be available.
- Filtration of exhaust from potent dry product handling areas and exhaust through HEPA filters, scrubbers, or other equivalent treatment methods prior to release outdoors may be required. Exhaust/return filters should be located as near to processing area as possible to reduce the length of potentially contaminated air ducts. For exhaust systems where the discharge contaminant is considered particularly hazardous, two banks of HEPA filters (Bag in /Bag out) in series should be considered to provide additional protection should the first filter fail.
- All filter banks should be provided with pressure differential indication gauges to indicate the filter dust loading and remaining life span of the filters.
- Appropriate monitoring and interlocking of HVAC with process equipment should be considered to maintain containment integrity and to control cross contamination and emissions.
- Performance of isolator protection (DP) should be monitored.
- Operators leaving the containment area should pass through air showers, to assist with removing dust particles from their garments.

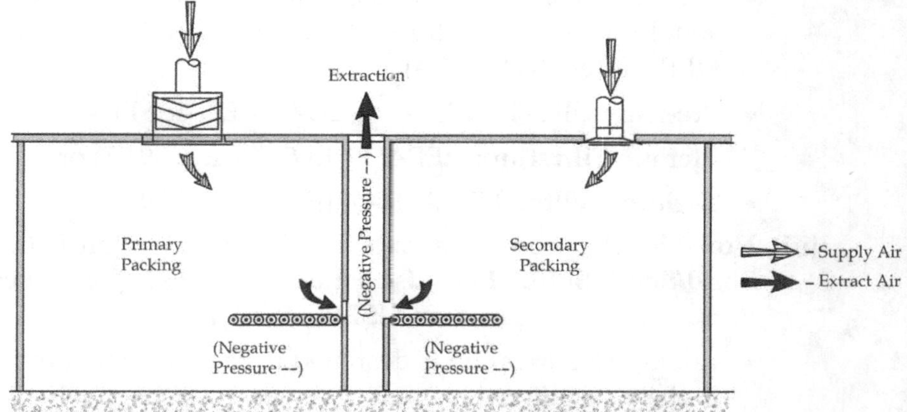

- Appropriate measures should be taken to prevent airflow from the primary packing area (through the conveyor "mouse hole") to the secondary packing area. This principle can be applied to other situations where containment from two sides is required.
- A typical mouse hole:

V. Design Acceptance Criteria:

- Acceptance criteria and limits should be defined during the design stage.
- Acceptable tolerances for all system parameters should be specified prior to commencing the physical installation.
- Critical and non-critical parameters should be determined by means of a risk analysis for all HVAC installation components, subsystems and controls.

VI. Check Points for Design Qualification Solid / Semi Solids / Liquids / Final API (Potent and Non Potent):

(i) What type of Air handling system is recommended in Non-Potent and Potent: Solid/Semi Solids/Liquids/ Final API facility? (Reference: ISPE HVAC)

- Processing room in the oral solid dosage form shall be capable of meeting Grade D (ISO 8) at rest for monitoring of particles.

(ii) What should be final filtration of in Non-Potent and Potent : Solid/Semi Solids/Liquids/ Final API facility?

- Air to Solid/Semi Solids/Liquids/ Final API area should be supplied through ceiling mounted terminal HEPA filters (H13/H14).
- **Pre-filters:** EU-10 & EU-9 or EU-7 or EU-6or EU-4
- **Plenum Filtration**: HEPA: H-13 **(Efficacy:** 99.95) or
- **Terminal Filter:** HEPA: H-14 (Efficacy: 99.995)

(iii) How is the room cascade designed in Non-Potent Solid/Semi Solids/Liquids/ Final API area? (Reference: WHOTRS 961, Annex-5 and ISPE- HVAC)

- Room pressurization is designed to cascade from area of highest cleanliness to areas of lower cleanliness.
- A pressure differential of 15 Pa is often used for achieving containment between two adjacent zones, but

pressure differentials of between 5 Pa and 20 Pa may be acceptable.

- Airlocks with different pressure cascade regimes include the cascade airlock, sink airlock and bubble airlock.

(iv) **What should be differential pressure between cubicles and corridor in Non-Potent: Solid/Semi Solids/Liquids/ Final API area?** (Reference: WHOTRS 961, Annex-5 and ISPE- HVAC)

- The corridor should be maintained at a higher pressure than the Cubicles and the cubicles at a higher pressure than atmospheric pressure.

(v) **What measure shall be taken when the multiple product are running at same time in** Non-**Potent and Potent : Solid/Semi Solids/Liquids/ Final API facility?** (Reference: WHOTRS 961, Annex-5 and ISPE- HVAC)

- Where different products are manufactured at the same time, in different areas or cubicles, in a multiproduct OSD manufacturing site, measures should be taken to ensure that dust cannot move from one cubicle to another.

(vi) **What should be designed of Potent: Solid/Semi Solids/Liquids/ Final API facility?** (Reference: WHOTRS 961, Annex-5 and ISPE- HVAC)

- Potent Drug facilities should be separate, dedicated facilities and should not form part of any other non-potent facility.
- They may be in the same building as another facility, but should be separated by a physical barrier and have separate entrances, staff facilities, air-handling systems, etc.
- A dedicated HVAC system is recommended for the controlled space where product is exposed.

(vii) **How the pressure cascada regime in maintained during the manufacturing of the product in processing area of Potent Solid/Semi Solids/Liquids/ Final API facility?** (Reference: WHOTRS 961, Annex-5 and ISPE- HVAC)

- Highly potent products should be manufactured under a pressure cascade regime that is negative relative to atmospheric pressure.

(viii) **How should be pressure between environment and of Potent Solid/Semi Solids/Liquids/ Final API facility?** (Reference: WHOTRS 961, Annex-5 and ISPE- HVAC)

- The facility should be maintained at a negative air pressure to the environment.

(ix) **How is the room cascade is designed in potent processing of Potent Solid/Semi Solids/Liquids/ Final API facility?** (Reference: WHOTRS 961, Annex-5 and ISPE- HVAC)

- Room air locks/anterooms are recommended for powder handling areas to provide a barrier that maintains a positive airflow differential with respect to the corridor and the processing room
- Airflow into de-gowning areas should be negative with respect to the corridor and processing area to contain particles shed from clothing.

(x) **What are Clean room requirements for permitted particles?** (Reference: Eudralex Annex-1)

Maximum permitted number of particles per m³ equal to or greater than the tabulated size				
Grade	At rest (b)		In Operation (a)	
	0.5µm	5µm	0.5µm	5µm
D	35,20,000	29000	Not defined (c)	Not defined (c)
For Grade D (at rest) the airborne particle classification is ISO 8.				

(xi) **What are the recommended limits for Microbiological Monitoring of clean area operation?** (Reference: Eudralex Annex-1)

Recommended limits for Microbiological Monitoring of Clean areas in operation:				
Grade	Air sample CFU /m³	Settle plates (dia. 90mm.) CFU/2 hrs.	Contact plates (dia.55mm) CFU per plate	Glove points (five fingers) CFU per glove
D	200	100	50	--
a. These are average values. b. Individual settle plates may be exposed for 30 or 1hr on justification.				

(xii) **Commission and Qualification and Maintenance:**

- Each clean area class should be specified as achieving the clean area classification under "as-built", "at-rest" or "operational" conditions.

- A room that is tested for an "operational" condition should be able to clean up to the "at-rest" clean area classification, after a short clean-up time. The clean-up time should be determined through validation.
- The "as-built" condition should relate to carrying out room classification tests on the bare room, without any equipment or personnel.
- The "at-rest" condition should relate to carrying out room classification tests with the normal production equipment in the room, but without any operators.
- The "operational" condition should relate to carrying out room classification tests with the normal production process with equipment operating, and the normal number of personnel present in the room.

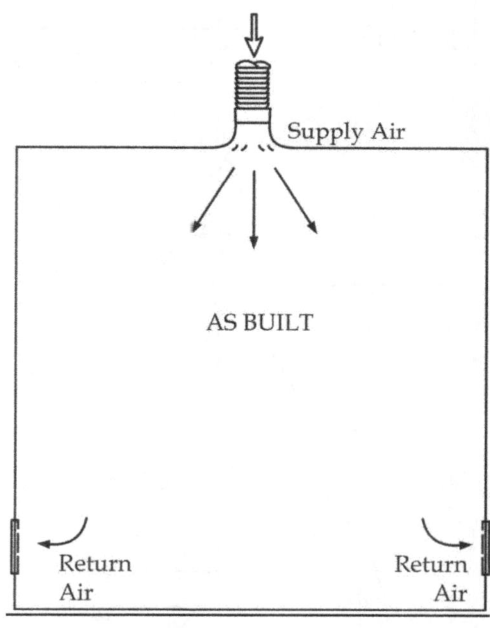

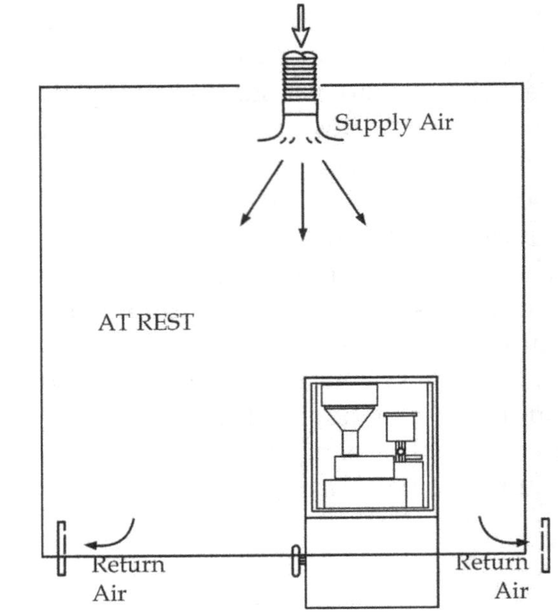

Supply Air
AT REST
Return
Air
Return
Air

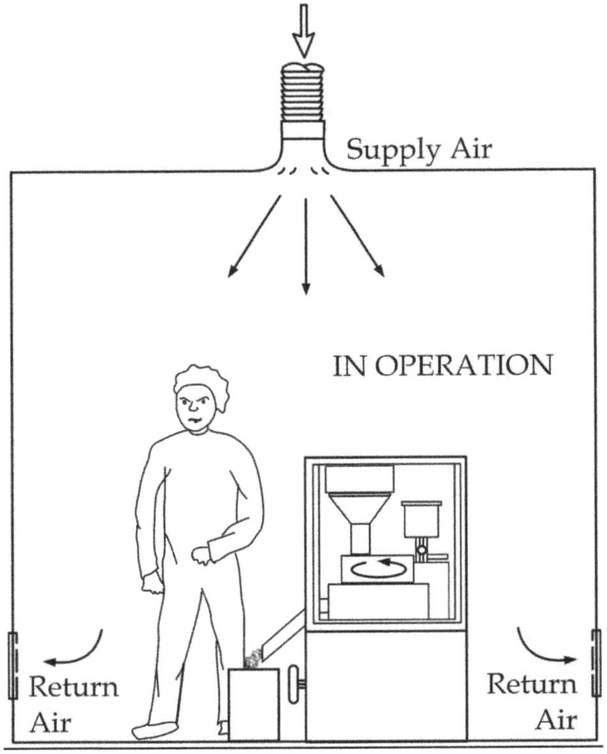

Supply Air
IN OPERATION
Return
Air
Return
Air

A. Installation Qualification:

- During Installation qualification, all the components and design meets the Design qualification.
- Commissioning shall involve the setting up, balancing, adjustment and testing of the entire HVAC system, to ensure that the system meets all the requirements of design.
- All critical instruments shall be calibrated.

B. Operational Qualification:

- There shall be no failure of fan at supply air, return air & exhaust air or dust extract system fan.
- Failure can cause a system imbalance, resulting in a pressure cascade malfunction with a resultant airflow reversal.
- Failure shall be addressed through Incident Management System.
- Design conditions and normal operating ranges shall be set during operational Qualification.
- Alert and action limits shall be established.

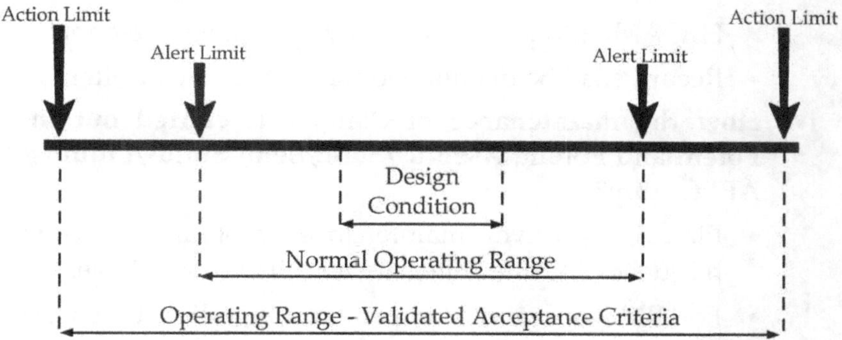

C. Performance Qualification:

Refer Aseptic Facilities.

22.2 Regular Check Points of HVAC System

i. Planned Preventive Maintenance for Non-Potent and Potent: Aseptic /Solid/Semi Solids/Liquids/ Final API facility:

- Each and every equipment and instrument which are used in formation of pharmaceutical product shall have approved calibration and planned preventive procedure.

- Planned Preventive Maintenance schedule shall be checked during audit.
- Calibration records of the instrument and equipment shall be checked with schedule and limit. E.g.: Temperature and RH sensor, pressure gauge etc.

ii. **Alarm Management for Non-Potent and Potent: Aseptic /Solid/Semi Solids/Liquids/ Final API facility:**

- Alarm management system shall be available and each and every alarm notification shall be timely investigation and recorded.
- Trend analysis for alarm generated shall be done.

iii. **HEPA filter for Non-Potent and Potent: Aseptic /Solid/Semi Solids/Liquids/ Final API facility:**

- Plan preventive maintenance program, records and frequency for filter integrity test shall be available.
- DOP is used for filter integrity test, which has integrity limit 0.01.
- Incident shall be raised and impact analysis shall be performed in the failure of filter integrity test.
- HEPA should be changed only by trained personnel.
- Record shall be maintained for destruction of filter.

iv. **How the maintenance of damper is carried out in Non-Potent and Potent: Aseptic /Solid/Semi Solids/Liquids/ Final API facility?**

- Plan preventive maintenance program, records and frequency for filter integrity test shall be available.
- For BMS operated damper working shall be checked for 0%, 50% and 100% opening.
- For manual handling damper checks can be done manual procedure.

v. **What is the procedure for Fumigation through HVAC system and which chemical are used in Non-Potent and Potent: Aseptic /Solid/Semi Solids/Liquids/ Final API facility?**

- Procedure and records for fumigation through HAVAC shall be available. Frequency and its chemical for fumigation shall be defined in procedure.

vi. How environment conditions are recorded in Non-Potent and Potent: Aseptic/Solid/Semi Solids/Liquids/ Final API facility?

- All graph or printout of the BMS or manual records shall be reviewed and any deviation to the environment monitoring shall be investigated.

vii. How the maintenance of BMS is carried out in Non-Potent and Potent: Aseptic /Solid/Semi Solids/Liquids/ Final API facility?

- Check the level of authorization and level of security in BMS system.
- Check the actual environment parameter with the validated parameter in the system.
- Check the preventive maintenance programme for BMS system.
- Check the audit trail system.
- Back up procedure shall be available for BMS data at different frequency and same shall be recorded.

viii. What is frequency for the requalification of HVAC?

- Requalification schedule shall be available.
- Frequency of requalification shall be based on risk assessment or any major change.

ix. How are air leakages checked in the area ?

- Procedure, frequency and record for air leakage from duct and area shall be available.
- Duct leakage is carried by soap test at the junction.

x. Verify the cleaning frequency of pre-filter, where it is cleaned and how it is destroyed?

- Procedure and frequency for cleaning of filter (Dry or wet) shall be available.
- Records for filter cleaning, destruction shall be available.
- Potent Drug filter shall be deactivated and send for destruction.

xi. Verify the cleaning frequency of dust collector filter, where it is cleaned and how it is destroyed?

- Procedure and frequency for cleaning of filter (Dry or wet) shall be available.

- Records for filter cleaning, destruction shall be available.
- Potent Drug filter shall be deactivated and send for destruction.

xii. **Verify the cleaning frequency of duct cleaning, and how it is cleaned?**

- Procedure and frequency for cleaning of duct shall be available.
- Manhole shall be available for cleaning of duct or robotic cleaning of duct shall be performed.
- Records for duct cleaning shall be available.

xiii. **Verify the cleaning frequency of heating and cooling coil and how it is cleaned?**

- Procedure for frequency cleaning of hot and cold coil with its record shall be available.
- Interlock system with cooler for cooling coil and interlock system with steam circulation or hot air circulation for hot coil shall be check during preventive maintenance.

22.3 Definition

- **Air-Handling Unit (AHU):** The air-handling unit serves to condition the air and provide the required air movement within a facility.
- **Airlock:** An enclosed space with two or more doors, which is interposed between two or more rooms, e.g. Differing classes of cleanliness, for the purpose of controlling the airflow between those rooms when they need to beentered.
- **Acceptance Criteria:** Measurable terms under which a test result considered acceptable.
- **Action limit:** The limit when the acceptance criteria of a particular parameter have been exceeded. Results outside these limits shall require specified action and investigation.
- **Alert limit:** The limit when the normal operating range of a particular parameter has been exceeded, indicating that corrective measures may be needed to prevent the action limit being reached.
- **As-built:** Condition where the installation is complete with all services connected and functioning but with no production equipment, materials or personnel present.

- **At-rest:** Condition where the installation is complete with equipment installed and operating in a manner agreed upon by the customer and supplier, but with no personnel present.
- **Clean Area (clean room):** An area (or room or zone) with defined environmental control of particulate and microbial contamination, constructed and used in such a way as to reduce the introduction, generation and retention of contaminants within the area.
- **Commissioning:** Commissioning is the documented process of verifying that the equipment and systems are installed according to specifications, placing the equipment into active service and verifying its proper action. Commissioning takes place at the conclusion of project construction but prior to validation.
- **Containment:** A process or device to contain product, dust or contaminants in one zone, preventing it from escaping to another zone.
- **Contamination :**The undesired introduction of impurities of a chemical or microbial nature, or of foreign matter, into or on to a starting material or intermediate, during production, sampling, packaging or repackaging, storage or transport.
- **Controlled Area:** An area within the facility in which specific environmental facility conditions and procedures are defined, controlled, and monitored to prevent degradation or cross-contamination of the product.
- **Critical Parameter or Component:** A processing parameter (such as temperature or relative humidity) that affects the quality of a product, or a component that may have a direct impact on the quality of the product.
- **Critical Quality Attribute (CQA):** A physical, chemical, biological or microbiological property or characteristic that should be within an appropriate limit, range or distribution to ensure the desired product quality.
- **Supply Air:** Supply air is a mixture of outdoor air and return air (re-circulated air) or 100% fresh air that is treated, conditioned, and supplied to the room through HVAC system.
- **Return Air:** Return air is air from the room that is re-circulated into the mixing chamber by the HVAC system in the area.

- **Exhaust Air:** Exhaust air is the air from the room that is exhausted from the building by the HVAC system in the area.
- **Supply Air Damper:** The supply dampers control the amount of air that will be re-circulated in the area.
- **Return Air Damper:** The return dampers control the amount of air that will be re-circulated in the area.
- **Exhaust Air Damper:** The exhaust air damper controls, the amount of air that is exhausted from the building. This damper's controls are often connected to outdoor air damper controls to provide a balance of outdoor air inflow and exhaust air outflow.
- **Air Flow Formula and Volume Calculation:**

$$\text{CFM} = \text{Duct area sq ft} \times \text{Velocity}$$

$$\text{Air Changes per Hours} = \frac{\text{CFM} \times 60}{\text{Cubic Feet}}$$

$$\text{CFM} = \frac{\text{Room Volume} \times \text{Air Changes per Hour}}{60}$$

- **Air Flow:** Air Flow is a measurement of the amount of air per unit of time that flows through a particular device. The amount of air can be measured by its volume or by its mass.

CHAPTER 23

Manufacturing Execution System (MES) in Pharmaceutical Industry

Introduction

- **MES** implementation **in two words: Execution and Integration**. MES software are tools designed to help a company to manage its manufacturing processes and inventory on shop. MES technology allows paper-documentation to be replaced with computerized records which can be accessed in real-time by all users, which helps to ensure **'Right-First-Time'** manufacturing and documentation. An MES gives real-time shop floor information.

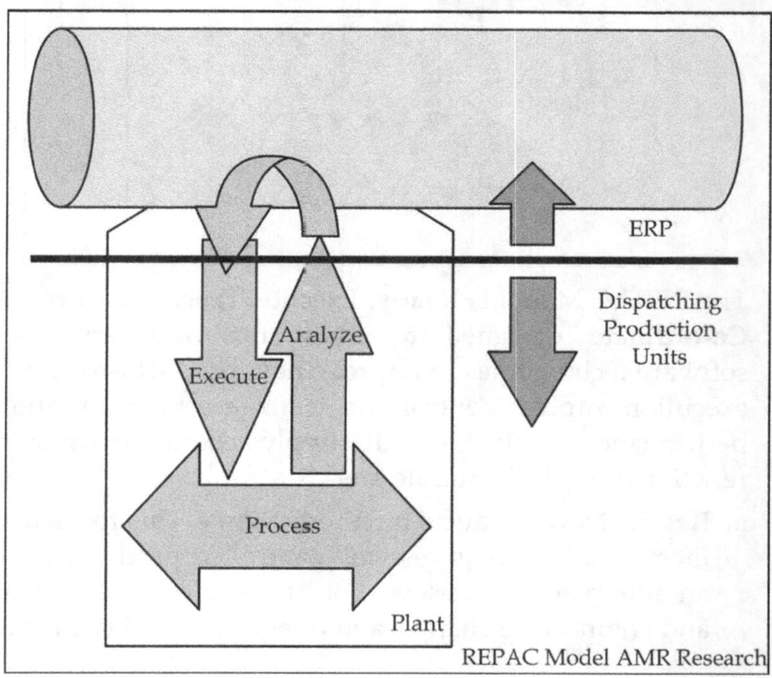

REPAC Model AMR Research

- MES **controls**, optimizes, and documents processes executed on the shop floor in full compliance with all the pharmaceutical requirements to increase security and reliability of the manufacturing process. MES are not isolated, but a core component of the entire supply chain IT architecture. In 1998, AMR created the REPAC Model and thus laid the foundations for the basic understanding of the necessity to use an MES.
- A Manufacturing Execution System is an electronic interface between personnel, equipment, automation, orders, logistics, equipment and batch record. The MES mediates between business administration (covering core functions such as sales and production planning or controlling) and the automation of the production process.

23.1 Overview of REPAC Model

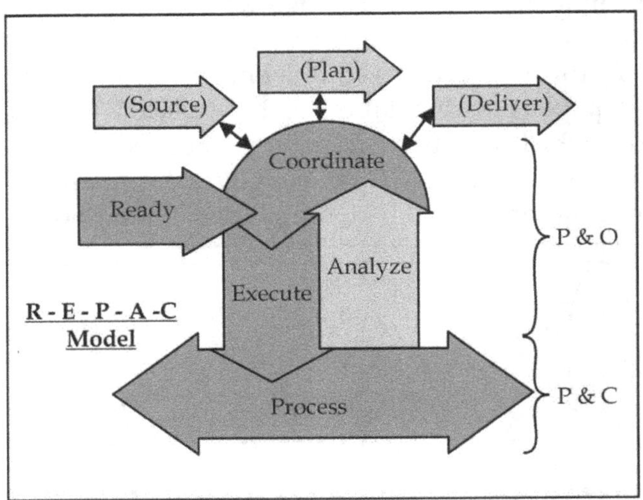

- The REPAC Model is **Ready, Execute, Process Control, Analyze, Co-ordinate** designed to assist manufacturers selecting n software technologies to improve new product production, order execution, process control and management, plant and product performance analysis, and supply chain coordination. Key function of REPAC module are:

  a. **Ready:** New Products for Production - This focus on Product lifecycles. This requires well controlled production processes, an automated, paperless process of new product introduction and engineering change, and integrated Quality Management.

b. **Execute:** Orders for Products- This process focuses on the execution of orders and processes such as personnel, equipment, and recording actual progress.

c. **Process:** Capability Control and Management – It focuses on the automation and control of Plant Systems which including MMI, SCADA, PLC, DCS and equipment with embedded controls.

d. **Analyze:** Plant and Product Performance- This step focuses on identifying and using key performance information to further improve the process in a number of areas such as: quality and production improvement.

e. **Coordinate:** Plant Internally Supply Chain and Equipment: This final step is responsible for constantly updating the plant's schedule so everyone knows the best thing to be doing each time they start a new task.

23.2 Over view of Three-Layer-Model

Manufacturing Execution Systems depends on Three-Layer-Model and consists three main activities in three groups of information:

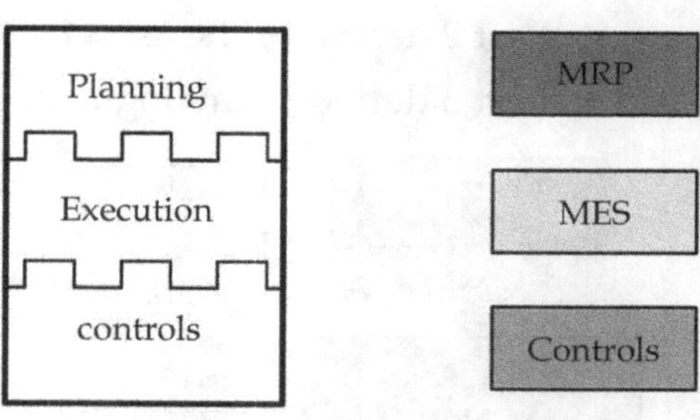

- **Plan Layer** – It is a top layer comprises of systems such as Enterprise Resource Planning (ERP), Manufacturing Resource Planning (MRPII), Material Requirements Planning (MRP), Capacity Requirements Planning (CRP) and Supply Chain Management (SCM).
- The **Execution Layer** acts as link between the control and planning layer. Communication between the execution and control layers occurs in real-time.
- **Control Layer: is established through devices and systems** such as programmable logic controllers (PLC), Supervisory Control and Data Acquisition (SCADA) and Man-Machine Interfaces (MMI). Information from these devises is sent in real-time to execution layer. Work, process and maintenance instructions are sent back.

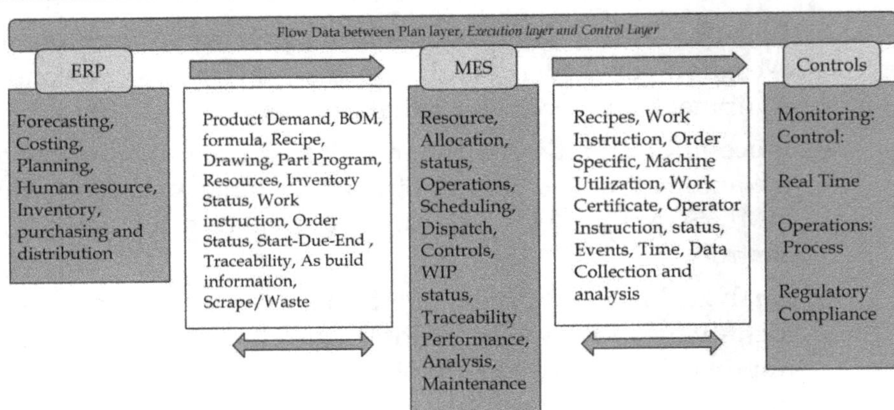

23.3 Overview of Standards ISA S95.00.01 / 02 / 03 for MES

- The ISA standard S95 focuses on the aspect of integration into IT environments and consists of three individual parts:
- Part 1 defines models for describing the distribution of tasks between ERP and MES systems (ISA-95.00.01) [1].
- Part 2 describes the associated data models (ISA-95.00.02) [2].
- Part 3 defines a catalogue of functions (ISA-95.00.03) [3].

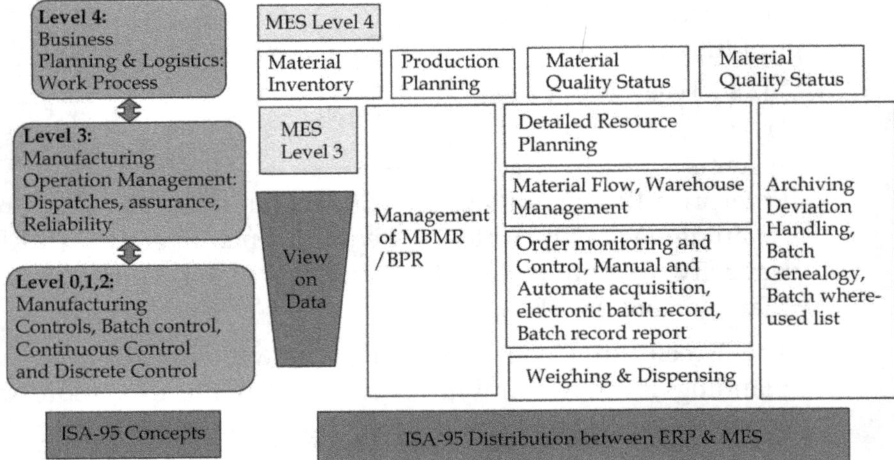

23.4 Systematic Planning Approach to MES Implementation in 14 stages

a. **Explore EMS:** Arrives as solution to ongoing problems or pain. Research into MES and desire to continue

b. **MES Project Feasibility:** Feasibility emerges with requirements definition and stakeholder involvement.

c. **Project Analysis:** Gap Analysis looks at current and future states and identifies a path and deliverables

d. **Make vs. Buy:** Data collection on available systems (OOB and build-to-suit)

e. **Choosing a Vendor:** Decision making tools such as AHP are employed to make a qualitative and quantitative analysis of the proposed solutions

f. **Statement of Work (SOW):** Collaboration between company and vendor on defining all aspects of project

g. **Gap Analysis:** Understanding of the discrepancies halting implementation of MES

h. **System Architecture :** Software and hardware design from specifications of MES

i. **Pilot Program:** Solidifies the functionalities desired within MES specific for the pilot program, and determines data collection methods.

j. **Implementation:** Implementation of all previously defined design, both high level and detailed

k. **Test Prototype MES:** Conference room pilot where stakeholders assign theoretical roles and 'move' product through the system.

l. **Verification and Validation**: Qualify direct and indirect benefits and check system has met desired levels of functionality.

m. **Full Scale Implementation:** All actions must be repeated for each product line and functionality.

n. **Monitor & Maintain:** Day-to-day operation is maintained and feature additions/subtractions managed and Ongoing for the lifecycle of MES

23.5 MES Functions

- MES should have function as per the standard S95:

Production Operations	Definition of production, Management of resources, Planning and execution of product manufacturing, Acquisition, documentation, and analysis of production
Product Management	Additional material master data, Definition of master batch record, Bill of material, Operations, Material flow in production, Review and approval workflow, Management of versions
Production management	Management of personnel and consideration of proper certification, Equipment management, e.g. container, scales, tanks, setup parts, workrooms, Management of material resources, Coordination with maintenance management, Management of future resource capabilities, Equipment management, ensuring the right status for usage (like cleaned, in use, calibration required), Electronic logbooks
Detailed production scheduling	Allocation of shop floor orders to machines, Comparison between actual and scheduled production, Monitoring of work centers and resources and Monitoring of order statuses
Production dispatching	Allocation of resources (personnel, equipment, material) to manufacturing orders, shop floor orders, Starting, stopping, interrupting and resuming of production order, Batch record execution, Performing assigned procedures and activities, Reacting to deviations, Throwing exceptions, Taking samples, Review and approval of batch record
Production data collection	Manual data acquisition, Automated data acquisition, Weighing and dispensing using scales, Calculation of new values based on formulas, Storing of production data in event or time context (trends), Acquisition of deviations, events and alarms
Production tracking	Electronic batch record report, Batch genealogy, Batch where-used list, Deviation handling, Tracking of all material movements, Process analysis, Statistical process control, Production performance analysis (KPIs, e.g. cycle times, resource utilization, equipment utilization)

23.6 Implementation Strategy

(i) **Regulatory Requirements:** An MES system for the pharmaceutical industry must functionally comply with the requirements of regulatory authorities in Europe, United States, GAMP 5, electronic signature and qualified to prove that all the requirements for the respective phase have been fulfilled and meets the regulatory requirement.

(ii) **Understanding MES Architectures:**

- **Enterprise Architecture:** Multiple production sites data from each sites is stored in the data center.
- **Redundant Architecture:** The redundant architecture will have a couple of Ignition servers in the data center.
- **Standard Architecture:** The simplest architecture for MES is to have a single server at a single site.

(iii) **Implementation in Phases:** The implementation should be carried **out in pilot phases**. In a pilot phase an existing, operational standard system (MES product) demonstrates the functions that are available or missing in the implementation. The findings can then be considered as improvement in the next phase, the implementation phase. Additional functions can be integrated in a roll-out version of software.

(iv) **Integration of All Key Users:** the key users should be integrated at a very early stage to analyzed its functionality. As soon as the pilot system is available, training courses should be held. In this phase, key users are just the right persons to make crucial contributions to improving the system or supported workflows.

(v) **Integrated Systems: The** MES is integrated into a comprehensive IT framework concept. There is a Unix-based system supporting materials planning, order creation and the entire supervisory control planning. So if recipes are changed in the MES the interface makes sure that the master data are automatically reconciled between MES, SAP and integrated system.

(vi) **Equipment Integration:** Equipment interfacing by means of PLCs enables the MES system to use automatically acquired data. The MES collects such operating data in a production database and places relevant data available for the manufacturing report.

(vii) **Focusing on Sophisticated System Configuration and Customization:** As MES systems are supposed to be flexible enough to adjust to the most versatile workflows, customization is necessary and wanted. The best way is to integrate process engineers, who are well-trained in defining master batch records, right from the start phase of the project.

(viii) **A Focus on Flexible Processes:** Any modification of the batch record or equipment's shall be documented and impact on the Master Batch Record shall be studied. Normal batch record data shall be collected continuously to compare to the stored recipe. Perodic verification of procedures and integrated process shall be done to ensure that all the workflows are correct. Transparency for the mapping and control of the complex material flow.

(ix) **The Reality of Electronic Documentation:** Periodic review for 21 CFR Part 11 compliances.

(x) **Manual and Automatic Sequences Alternating :**

- The automated sequences are first filed in the DCS recipe system and transferred to the MES. The MES then links these automated sub functions to the manual operations and consistency checks.
- The MES handles all the manual sequences and triggers the automated procedures in the DCS. On execution of automated sequences the DCS returns the result parameters to the MES. As the controlling system, the MES continually displays the current status of all processes including DCS. On completion of a manufacturing stage, the MES generates complete associated documentation.

CHAPTER 24

Pharmaceutical Drug Master File

Introduction

A DMF is required to supply bulk materials to the United States which provides confidential detailed information about facilities, processes, or articles used in the manufacturing, processing, packaging, and storing of one or more human drugs. However, the information contained in a DMF may be used to support, but not a substitute for an Investigational New Drug Application (IND), a New Drug Application (NDA), an Abbreviated New Drug Application (ANDA), another DMF, an Export Application, or related documents.

I. SUBMISSIONS TO DRUG MASTER FILES:

The DMF must be in the English language with date and consecutively number on each page. DMF submission contents transmittal letter, administrative information about the submission, and the specific information.

A. Transmittal Letters: Includes Original submission and Amendments

A.1 Original Submissions

- Identification of submission: Original, the type of DMF as classified in Section III, and its subject.
- Identification of the applications, if known, that the DMF is intended to support, including the name and address of each sponsor, applicant, or holder, and all relevant document numbers.
- Signature of the holder or the authorized representative.
- Typewritten name and title of the signer.

A.2 Amendments

- Identification of submission: Amendment, the DMF number, type of DMF, and the subject of the amendment.
- A description of the purpose of submission, e.g., update, revised formula, or revised process.
- Signature of the holder or the authorized representative.

Typewritten name and title of the signer.

B. Administrative Information: Includes Original submission and Amendments

B.1 Original Submissions

- Names and addresses of the following: DMF holder, Corporate headquarters, Manufacturing /processing facility, Contact for FDA correspondence. Agent(s), if any:
- The specific responsibilities of each person listed in any of the categories in Section.
- Statement of commitment.
- A signed statement by the holder certifying that the DMF is current and that the DMF holder will comply with the statements made in it.

B.2 Amendments

- Name of DMF holder.
- DMF number.
- Name and address for correspondence.
- Affected section and/or page numbers of the DMF.
- The name and address of each person whose IND, NDA, ANDA, DMF, or Export Application relies on the subject of the amendment for support.
- The number of each IND, NDA, ANDA, DMF, and Export Application that relies on the subject of the amendment for support, if known.
- Particular items within the IND, NDA, ANDA, DMF, and Export Application that are affected, if known.

II. TYPES OF DRUG MASTER FILE AND ITS CONTENTS:

There are five types of Drug Master Files.

- **Type I: Manufacturing Site, Facilities, Operating Procedures, and Personnel: The** DMF should outside the United states to describe the manufacturing site, equipment capabilities, and operational layout.
- **Type II: Drug Substance, Drug Substance Intermediate, and Material Used in Their Preparation, or Drug Product :** limited to a single drug intermediate, drug substance, drug product, or type of material used in their preparation.
- **Drug Substance Intermediates, Drug Substances, and Material Used in Their Preparation:** Summarize all significant steps in the manufacturing and controls of the drug intermediate or substance.
- **Drug Product:** *Content of the Chemistry, Manufacturing, and Controls, Documentation for the Manufacture of and Controls for Drug Products and Samples and Analytical Data for Methods Validation.*
- **Type III: Packaging Material:**
- The names of the suppliers or fabricators of the components. used in preparing the packaging material and the acceptance specifications.
- Data supporting the acceptability of the packaging material for its intended use.
- Toxicological data on these materials.
- **Type IV : Excipient, Colorant, Flavor, Essence, or Material Used in Their Preparation:**
- Each additive should be identified and characterized by its method of manufacture, release specifications, and testing methods.
- Toxicological data on these materials would be included under this type of DMF, if not otherwise available by cross reference to another document.
- **Type V: FDA Accepted Reference Information:**
- Miscellaneous information, duplicate information, or information that should be included in one of the other types of DMF's.

III. GENERAL INFORMATION AND SUGGESTIONS:

- **Environmental Assessment:** Type II, Type III, and Type IV DMF's should contain a commitment by the firm that its facilities will be operated in compliance with applicable environmental laws.
- **Stability:** Stability study design, data, interpretation, and other information should be submitted.

IV. FORMAT, ASSEMBLY, AND DELIVERY:

An original and duplicate are to be submitted for all DMF submissions: Drug Master File holders and their agents/representatives should retain a complete reference copy that is identical to, and maintained in the same chronological order as, their submissions to FDA.

- The original and duplicate copies must be collated, fully assembled, and individually jacketed: Each volume of a DMF should, in general, be no more than 2 inches thick. For multivolume submissions, number each volume.
- U.S. standard paper size (8-1/2 by 11 inches) is preferred.

V. DRUG MASTER FILE SUBMISSIONS AND CORRESPONDENCE SHOULD BE ADDRESSED AS FOLLOWS:

Drug Master File Staff

Food and Drug Administration

5901-B Ammendale Rd.

Beltsville, MD 20705-1266

VI. AUTHORIZATION TO REFER TO A DRUG MASTER FILE

Letter of Authorization to FDA: Before FDA can review DMF information in support of an application, the DMF holder must submit in duplicate to the DMF a letter of authorization permitting FDA to reference the DMF.The letter of authorization should include the following:

The date.

Name of DMF holder.

DMF number.

Name of person(s) authorized to incorporate information in the DMF by reference.

Specific product(s) covered by the DMF.

Submission date(s)

Section numbers and/or page numbers to be referenced.

Statement of commitment that the DMF is current and that the DMF holder will comply with the statements made in it.

Signature of authorizing official.

Typed name and title of official authorizing reference to the DMF.

Copy to Applicant, Sponsor, or Other Holder: The holder should also send a copy of the letter of authorization to the affected applicant, sponsor, or other holder who is authorized to incorporate by reference the specific information contained in the DMF.

VII. PROCESSING AND REVIEWING POLICIES:

A. Policies Related to Processing Drug Master Files:

- Public availability of the information and data in a DMF
- An original DMF submission will be examined on receipt to determine whether it meets minimum requirements for format and content. If the submission is administratively acceptable, FDA will acknowledge its receipt and assign it a DMF number.(If the submission is administratively incomplete or inadequate, it will be returned to the submitter with a letter of explanation from the Drug Master File Staff, and it will not be assigned a DMF number).

B. Drug Master File Review:

- A DMF IS NEVER APPROVED OR DISAPPROVED. : The agency will review information in a DMF only when an IND sponsor, an applicant for an NDA, ANDA, or Export Application, or another DMF holder incorporates material in the DMF by reference.

VIII. HOLDER OBLIGATIONS:

- Any change or addition, including a change in authorization related to specific customers, should be submitted in duplicate and adequately cross referenced to previous submission(s). The reference should include the date(s), volume(s), section(s), and/or page number(s) affected.

A. Notice Required for Changes to a Drug Master File:

B. Listing of Persons Authorized To Refer to a Drug Master File:

- A DMF is required to contain a complete list of persons authorized to incorporate information in the DMF by reference. The holder should update the list in the annual update. The updated list should contain the holder's name, DMF number, and the date of the update. The update should identify by name (or code) the information that each person is authorized to incorporate and give the location of that information by date, volume, and page number.
- Any person whose authorization has been withdrawn during the previous year should be identified under a suitable caption.
- If the list is unchanged on the anniversary date, the DMF holder should also submit a statement that the list is current.

C. Annual Update: The holder should provide an annual report on the anniversary date of the original submission. Identify all changes and additional information incorporated into the DMF since the previous annual report on the subject matter of the DMF.

D. Appointment of an Agent: When an agent is appointed, the holder should submit a signed letter of appointment to the DMF giving the agent's name, address, and scope of responsibility.

E. Transfer of Ownership: To transfer ownership of a DMF to another party, the holder should so notify FDA and authorized persons in writing. The letter should include the following:

- Name of transferee
- Address of transferee
- Name of responsible official of transferee
- Effective date of transfer
- Signature of the transferring official
- Typewritten name and title of the transferring official.

- The new holder should submit a letter of acceptance of the transfer and an update of the information contained in the DMF, where appropriate. Any change relating to the new ownership (e.g., plant location and methods) should be included.

IX. MAJOR REORGANIZATION OF A DRUG MASTER FILE:

- A holder who plans a major reorganization of a DMF is encouraged to submit a detailed plan of the proposed changes and request its review by the Drug Master File Staff. The staff should be given sufficient time to comment and provide suggestions before a major reorganization is undertaken.

X. CLOSURE OF A DRUG MASTER FILE:

- A holder who wishes to close a DMF should submit a request to the Drug Master File Staff stating the reason for the closure.

XI. SUBMISSION PROCESS OF DRUG PRODUCT:

Submission	**India**	**EU**	**USA**
Application	MAA	MAA	ANDA
Department Certification	**NA**	**NA**	Required
No. of copies	**1**	**1**	**3**
Approval time line	12 Month	12 Month	18 Month
CTD	eCTD	eCTD	eCTD

CHAPTER 25

Common Technical Document in Regulatory Filing

Introduction

- CTD is an internationally agreed "well-structured common format" to assemble all the Quality, Safety and Efficacy information in a common format. It consist of unambiguous and transparent information to review applicant content.
- The Common Technical Document is organized into five modules. Module 1 is region specific. Modules 2, 3, 4, and 5 are intended to be common for all regions.he CTD became the mandatory format for new drug applications in the EU and Japan, and the strongly recommended format of choice for NDAs submitted to the FDA.

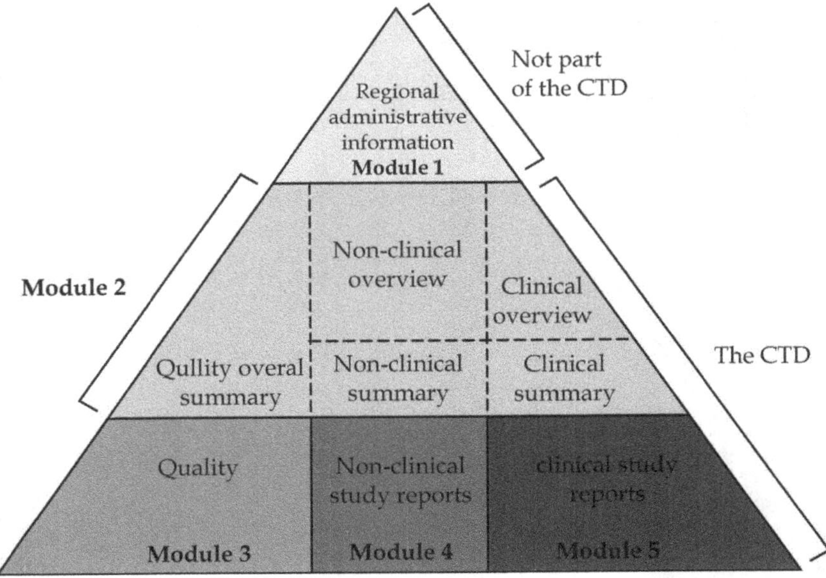

25.1 Organization of the Common Technical Document

- Module1 is for administrative information and prescribing information of the region with documentation. Module 2 contains the CTD summaries and begin with a general introduction to the drug, including its pharmacological class, mode of action and proposed clinical use. Module 2 also provide the overall summary of the 'quality' information provided, the non-clinical overview and the clinical overview, as well as the non-clinical written summaries and the tabulated summaries, and the clinical summary.
- Module 3 contains information on quality topics, module 4 contains the nonclinical study reports and module 5 contains the clinical study reports.

➢ **Module 1: Administrative Information and Prescribing Information**

- Table of Contents of the Submission Including Module 1.
- Documents Specific to Each Region (for example, application forms, prescribing information).

➢ **Module 2: Common Technical Document Summaries**

- Common Technical Document Table of Contents (Modules 2-5)
- CTD Introduction

A. DRUG SUBSTANCE (NAME AND MANUFACTURER)

- General Information (name, manufacturer)
- Manufacture (name, manufacturer)
- Characterisation (name, manufacturer)
- Control of Drug Substance (name, manufacturer)
- Reference Standards or Materials (name, manufacturer)
- Container Closure System (name, manufacturer)
- Stability (name, manufacturer)

B. DRUG PRODUCT (NAME, DOSAGE FORM)

- Description and Composition of the Drug Product (name, dosage form)
- Pharmaceutical Development (name, dosage form)
- Manufacture (name, dosage form)

- Control of Excipients (name, dosage form).
- Control of Drug Product (name, dosage form).
- Reference Standards or Materials (name, dosage form).
- Container Closure System (name, dosage form).
- Stability (name, dosage form).
    - Quality Overall Summary
    - Nonclinical Overview
- General Aspects.
- Content and Structural Format.

Nonclinical Written and Tabulated Summaries

- Nonclinical Written Summaries
- Introduction
- General Presentation Issues

A. Introduction

B. Pharmacology Written Summary

- Brief Summary
- Primary Pharmacodynamics
- Secondary Pharmacodynamics
- Safety Pharmacology
- Pharmacodynamic Drug Interactions
- Discussion and Conclusions
- Tables and Figures

C. Pharmacology Tabulated Summary

D. Pharmacokinetics Written Summary

- Brief Summary
- Methods of Analysis
- Absorption
- Distribution
- Metabolism (interspecies comparison
- Excretion
- Pharmacokinetic Drug Interactions
- Other Pharmacokinetic Studies
- Discussion and Conclusions
- Tables and Figures

E. Pharmacokinetics Tabulated Summary

F. Toxicology Written Summary

- Brief Summary
- Single-Dose Toxicity
- Repeat-Dose Toxicity (including supportive toxicokinetics evaluation)
- Genotoxicity
- Carcinogenicity (including supportive toxicokinetics evaluations)
- Reproductive and Developmental Toxicity (including range-finding studies and supportive toxicokinetics evaluations
- Local Tolerance
- Other Toxicity Studies (if available)
- Discussion and Conclusions
- Tables and Figures

G. Toxicology Tabulated Summary

- **Clinical Overview**

  A. Preamble

  B. Table of Contents

  C. Detailed Discussion of Content of the Clinical Overview Sections

  - Product Development Rationale
  - Overview of Biopharmaceutics
  - Overview of Clinical Pharmacology
  - Overview of Efficacy
  - Overview of Safety
  - Benefits and Risks Conclusions
  - Literature References

- **Clinical Summary**

  A. Preamble

  B. Table of Contents

  C. Detailed Guidance on Sections of the Clinical Summary

i. **Summary of Biopharmaceutic Studies and Associated Analytical Methods**
   - Background and Overview
   - Summary of Results of Individual Studies
   - Comparison and Analyses of Results Across Studies
   - Appendix

ii. **Summary of Clinical Pharmacology Studies**
   - Background and Overview
   - Summary of Results of Individual Studies
   - Comparison and Analyses of Results Across Studies
   - Special Studies
   - Appendix

iii. **Summary of Clinical Efficacy**
   - Background and Overview of Clinical Efficacy
   - Summary of Results of Individual Studies
   - Comparison and Analyses of Results Across Studies
     a. Study Populations
     b. Comparison of Efficacy Results of all Studies
     c. Comparison of Results in Sub-populations
   - Analysis of Clinical Information Relevant to Dosing Recommendations
   - Persistence of Efficacy and/or Tolerance Effects
   - Appendix

- **Summary of Clinical Safety**

  A. **Exposure to the Drug**
     - Overall Safety Evaluation Plan and Narratives of Safety Studies
     - Overall Extent of Exposure
     - Demographic and Other Characteristics of Study Population

B. **Adverse Events**
- Analysis of Adverse Events
- Narratives

C. **Clinical Laboratory Evaluations**

D. **Vital Signs, Physical Findings, and Other Observations Related to Safety**

E. **Safety in Special Groups and Situations**
- Intrinsic Factors
- Extrinsic Factors
- Drug Interactions
- Use in Pregnancy and Lactation
- Overdose
- Drug Abuse
- Withdrawal and Rebound
- Effects on Ability to Drive or Operate Machinery or Impairment of Mental Ability

F. **Post-marketing Data**

G. **Appendix**

iv. **Literature References**

v. **Synopsesof Individual Studies**

➢ **Module 3: Quality**
- Table of Contents of Module 3
- Body of Data

A. DRUG SUBSTANCE (NAME, MANUFACTURER)

a. **General Information (name, manufacturer)**
- Nomenclature (name, manufacture)
- Structure (name, manufacturer)

b. **General Properties (name, manufacturer)**
- Manufacturer(s) (name, manufacturer)
- Description of Manufacturing Process and Process Controls (name, manufacturer)
- Control of Materials (name, manufacturer)
- Controls of Critical Steps and Intermediates (name, manufacturer)

- Process Validation and/or Evaluation (name, manufacturer)
- Manufacturing Process Development (name, manufacturer)

c. **Characterization (name, manufacturer)**
- Elucidation of Structure and other Characteristics (name, manufacturer)
- Impurities (name, manufacturer)

d. **Control of Drug Substance (name, manufacturer)**
- Specification (name, manufacturer)
- Analytical Procedures (name, manufacturer)
- Validation of Analytical Procedures (name, manufacturer)
- Batch Analyses (name, manufacturer)
- Justification of Specification (name, manufacturer)

e. **Reference Standards or Materials (name, manufacture)**

f. **Container Closure System (name, manufacturer)**

g. **Stability (name, manufacturer)**
- Stability Summary and Conclusions (name, manufacturer)
- Post-approval Stability Protocol and Stability Commitment (name, manufacturer)
- Stability Data (name, manufacturer)

B. **DRUG PRODUCT (NAME, DOSAGE FORM)**

a. **Description and Composition of the Drug Product (name, dosage form)**

b. **Pharmaceutical Development (name, dosage form)**

i. **Components of the Drug Product (name, dosage form)**
- Drug Substance (name, dosage form)
- Excipients (name, dosage form

ii. **Drug Product (name, dosage form)**
- Formulation Development (name, dosage form)

- Overages (name, dosage form)
- Physicochemical and Biological Properties (name, dosage form)

iii. **Manufacturing Process Development (name, dosage form)**

iv. **Container Closure System (name, dosage form)**

v. **Microbiological Attributes (name, dosage form)**

vi. **Compatibility (name, dosage form)**

c. **Manufacture (name, dosage form)**

- Manufacturer(s) (name, dosage form)
- Batch Formula (name, dosage form)
- Description of Manufacturing Process and Process Controls (name, dosage form)
- Controls of Critical Steps and Intermediates (name, dosage form)
- Process Validation and/or Evaluation (name, dosage form)

d. **Control of Excipients (name, dosage form)**

- Specifications (name, dosage form)
- Analytical Procedures (name, dosage form)
- Validation of Analytical Procedures (name, dosage form)
- Justification of Specifications (name, dosage form)
- Excipients of Human or Animal Origin (name, dosage form)
- Novel Excipients (name, dosage form)

e. **Control of Drug Product (name, dosage form)**

- Specification(s) (name, dosage form)
- Analytical Procedures (name, dosage form)
- Validation of Analytical Procedures (name, dosage form)
- Batch Analyses (name, dosage form)
- Characterisation of Impurities (name, dosage form)
- Justification of Specification(s) (name, dosage form)

C. REFERENCE STANDARDS OR MATERIALS (NAME, DOSAGE FORM)

D. CONTAINER CLOSURE SYSTEM (NAME, DOSAGE FORM)

E. STABILITY (NAME, DOSAGE FORM)

- Stability Summary and Conclusion (name, dosage form)
- Post-approval Stability Protocol and Stability Commitment (name, dosage form)
- Stability Data (name, dosage form)
- Literature References

➢ **Module 4: Nonclinical Study Reports**

- Table of Contents of Module 4
- Study Reports
- Literature References

➢ **Module 5: Clinical Study Reports**

- Preamble
- Detailed **Organisation of Clinical Study Reports and Related Information in Module**

A. Table of Contents of Module 5

B. Tabular Listing of All Clinical Studies

C. Clinical Study Reports

i. **Reports of Biopharmaceutic Studies**
   - Bioavailability (BA) Study Reports
   - Comparative BA and Bioequivalence (BE) Study Reports
   - *In Vitro – In Vivo* Correlation Study Reports
   - Reports of Bioanalytical and Analytical Methods for Human Studies

ii. **Reports of Studies Pertinent to Pharmacokinetics Using Human Biomaterials**
   - Plasma Protein Binding Study Reports
   - Reports of Hepatic Metabolism and Drug Interaction Studies
   - Reports of Studies Using Other Human Biomaterials

iii. **Reports of Human Pharmacokinetic (PK) Studies**
- Healthy Subject PK and Initial Tolerability Study Reports
- Patient PK and Initial Tolerability Study Reports
- Intrinsic Factor PK Study Reports
- Extrinsic Factor PK Study Reports
- Population PK Study Reports

iv. **Reports of Human Pharmacodynamic (PD) Studies**
- Healthy Subject PD and PK/PD Study Reports
- 5.3.4.2 Patient PD and PK/PD Study Reports

v. **Reports of Efficacy and Safety Studies**
- Study Reports of Controlled Clinical Studies Pertinent to the Claimed
- Indication
- Study Reports of Uncontrolled Clinical Studies
- Reports of Analyses of Data from More than One Study
- Other Study Reports

vi. **Reports of Post-Marketing Experience**

vii. **Case Report Forms and Individual Patient Listings**
- **Literature References**

25.2 Electronic Common Technical Document (eCTD)

Electronic common technical document is called as eCTD. The granularity of the paper and electronic submissions is equivalent, although if a paper submission is updated to be an electronic submission, some changes in granularity could be introduced to facilitate on-going lifecycle management. In an electronic submission, a new file starts at the same point at which in a paper submission, a tabdivides the documents.

CHAPTER 26

European Union Marketing Authorization

Introduction

The European Union,(EU) consisting of 27 Member States. There are three procedures for submitting a Marketing Authorization Application (MAA) in the EU:

a. The mutual recognition procedure (MRP);

b. The decentralized (DCP) and

c. The centralized procedure (CP).

- The submission strategy will depend on the nature of the product, the target indication(s), the history of the product, and the marketing plan The centralized procedure (CP) leads to approval of the product in all 27 EU member states. Submission of one Marketing Authorization Application (MAA) thus leads to one assessment process and one authorization that allows access to the market of the entire EU. When using the mutual recognition procedure (MRP); or decentralized (DCP), the applicant must select which and how many EU member states in which to seek approval. In the case of an MRP, the applicant must initially receive national approval in one EU member state. This will be the so-called reference member state (RMS) for the mutual recognition procedure (MRP). Then, the applicant seeks approval for the product in other EU member states, the so-called concerned member states (CMS) in a second step: the mutual recognition process. For the decentralized (DCP), the applicant will approach all chosen member states at the same time. To do so, the applicant will identify the reference member state (RMS) that will assess the submitted Marketing Authorization Application (MAA) and provide the other selected member states with the conclusions und results of the assessment. In principle, the applicant can choose any EU member state as reference member state (RMS); however, in almost all member states the applicants need to send a request for a time slot when they will be allowed to submit the application. Depending on the agency selected as reference member state (RMS), the interval between submission of the request to the actual submission date can be two years or longer.

A. Mutual Recognition Procedure (MRP):

- The **mutual-recognition procedure**, whereby a marketing authorization granted in one Member State can be recognized in other EU countries. The mutual recognition procedure is to be used in order to obtain marketing authorizations in several Member States where the medicinal product in question has received a marketing authorization in any Member State at the time of application. In the mutual recognition procedure, the reference member state (RMS)has already issued a national marketing authorisation. The applicant can decide in which other Member States it would like to have its veterinary medicinal product authorised; in those countries an application for marketing authorisation must be submitted. On the basis of the evaluation report of the reference member state (RMS), the other Member States are asked to recognise its marketing authorisation including the Summary of Product Characteristics (SPC), package leaflet and packaging texts.

a. Steps involved in the mutual recognition procedure

- The mutual recognition procedure is divided in the following steps:
- National validation by the reference Member State (not further described here)
- Preparation or update of assessment report by reference Member State (90 days)
- Validation by the concerned Member States
- Approval by the concerned Member States (90 days)
- Discussion at the coordination group level, if needed
- National Marketing Authorisation step

b. Flow chart for the Mutual Recognition Procedure

THE MUTUAL RECOGNITION PROCEDURE	
Approx. 90 days before submission to CMS	Applicant requests RMS to update Assessment Report (AR) and allocate procedure number.
Day -14	Applicant submits the dossier to concerned member states (CMS). reference member state (RMS) circulates the AR including Summary of Product Characteristics (SPC), PL and labelling to concerned member states (CMS). Validation of the application in the concerned member states (CMS)
Day 0	reference member state (RMS) starts the procedure
Day 50	concerned member states (CMS) send their comments to the reference member state (RMS) and applicant
Day 60	Applicant sends the response document to concerned member states (CMS) and reference member state (RMS)
Until Day 68	Reference member state (RMS) circulates their assessment of the response document to concerned member states (CMS)
Day 75	concerned member states (CMS) send their remaining comments to reference member state (RMS and applicant. A break-out session can be organised between day 73 – 80).
Day 85	concerned member states (CMS) send any remaining comments to reference member state (RMS) and applicant.
Day 90	concerned member states (CMS) notify reference member state (RMS and applicant of final position (and in case of negative position also the CMD (Coordination group for mutual recognition and decentralized procedure for human medicinal products) secretariat of the EMEA). • If consensus is reached, the reference member state (RMS) closes the procedure. • If consensus is not reached, the points for disagreement submitted by concerned member states (CMS) are referred to CMD (Coordination group for mutual recognition and decentralised procedure for human medicinal products)) by the reference member state (RMS) within 7 days after Day 90.

Contd...

THE MUTUAL RECOGNITION PROCEDURE	
Day 150	For procedures referred to CMD (Coordination group for mutual recognition and decentralised procedure for human medicinal products) • If consensus is reached at the level of CMD (Coordination group for mutual recognition and decentralised procedure for human medicinal products) the reference member state (RMS) closes the procedure. • If consensus is not reached at the level of CMD (Coordination group for mutual recognition and decentralised procedure for human medicinal products) the reference member state (RMS) refers the matter to CHMP for arbitration
5 days after close of Procedure	Applicant sends high quality national translations of Summary of Product Characteristics (SPC), PL and labelling to concerned member states (CMS) and reference member state (RMS).
30 days after close of Procedure	Granting of national marketing authorisations in the concerned member states (CMS) subject to submission of acceptable translations.

B. Decentralised Procedure:

- The **decentralised procedure**, whereby a medicine that has not yet been authorised in the EU can be simultaneously authorised in several EU Member States. The decentralised procedure is to be used in order to obtain marketing authorisations in several Member States where the medicinal product in question has not yet received a marketing authorisation in any Member State at the time of application. The Decentralised procedure can be used to obtain marketing authorisation in several Member States if the applicant does not have marketing authorisation for the relevant veterinary medicinal product in any country. The applicant requests one country to become the Reference Member State (RMS) in the procedure while submitting an application for marketing authorisation in all countries simultaneously .The Decentralised procedure has two evaluation phases. In the first evaluation round (120 days), the applicant has the possibility to submit additional data/studies after expiry of a clock-stop period. The second evaluation round lasts 90 days and is comparable to an

MRP. In principle, the concerned Member States accept the evaluation of the Reference Member State (RMS, unless there are serious objections that can be considered a potentially serious risk for the health of man or animal or for the environment.

a. Steps involved in the Decentralised procedure

The decentralised procedure is divided in five steps:

- Validation step
- Assessment step I
- Assessment step II
- Discussion at the coordination group level, if needed
- National Marketing Authorisation step

b. Flow Chart of the Decentralised Procedure

Decentralised Procedure	
Pre-procedural Step	
Before Day -14	Applicant discussions with reference member state (RMS),reference member state (RMS) allocates procedure number. Creation in CTS.
Day –14	Submission of the dossier to the reference member state (RMS) and concerned member states (CMS). Validation of the application –.
Assessment step I	
Day 0	reference member state (RMS) starts the procedure
Day 70	reference member state (RMS) forwards the Preliminary Assessment Report (PrAR),SPC , PL and labelling to the concerned member states (CMS)
Until Day 100	concerned member states (CMS) send their comments to the reference member state (RMS)
Until Day 105	Consultation between reference member state (RMS) and concerned member states (CMS) and applicant. If consensus not reached RMS stops the clock to allow applicant to supplement the dossier and respond to the questions.
Clock-off period	Applicant may send draft responses to the reference member state (RMS) and agrees the date with the reference member state (RMS) for submission of the final response. Applicant sends the final response document to the reference member state (RMS) and concerned member states (CMS) within a recommended period of 3 months, which could be extended if justified

Contd...

Decentralised Procedure	
Day 106	Valid submission of the response of the applicant received reference member state (RMS) restarts the procedure.
Day 106 – 120	reference member state (RMS)updates Preliminary Assessment Report (PrAR) to prepare Draft Assessment Report (DAR) draft Summary of Product Characteristics (SPC), draft labelling and draft PIL to concerned member states (CMS)
Day 120	reference member state (RMS) may close procedure if consensus reached. Proceed to national 30 days step for granting MA.
Assessment step II	
Day 120 (Day 0)	If consensus not reached reference member state (RMS) sends the Draft Assessment Report (DAR), draft SPC, draft labelling and draft PIL to concerned member states (CMS)
Day 145 (Day 25)	CMSs sends final comments to reference member state (RMS)
CMSs sends final comments to RMS **Day 150 (Day 30)**	reference member state (RMS) may close procedure if consensus reached. Proceed to national 30 days step for granting MA
Until 180 (Day 60)	If consensus is not reached by day 150, reference member state (RMS) to communicate outstanding issues with applicant, receive any additional clarification and prepare a short report for discussion at Coordination Group
Until Day 205 (Day85)	Breakout Group of involved Member States reaches consensus on the matter
Day 210 (Day 90)	Closure of the procedure including concerned member states (CMS) approval of assessment report, Summary of Product Characteristics (SPC), labelling and PIL, or referral to Co-ordination group. Proceed to national 30 days step for granting MA.
Day 210 (at the latest)	If consensus was not reached at day 210, points of disagreement will be referred to the Co-ordination group for resolution
Day 270 (at the latest)	Final position adopted by Co-ordination Group with referral to CHMP/CVMP for arbitration in case of unsolved disagreement
National step	
Day 110/125/155/215/275	Applicant sends high quality national translations of Summary of Product Characteristics (SPC), labelling and PIL to concerned member states (CMS and reference member state (RMS)

Contd...

Decentralised Procedure	
Day 135/150/180/240	Granting of national marketing authorisation in reference member state (RMS) and concerned member states (CMS) if no referral to the Co-ordination group. (National Agencies will adopt the decision and will issue the marketing authorisation subject to submission of acceptable translations).
Day 300	Granting of national marketing authorisation in reference member state (RMS) and concerned member states (CMS)if positive conclusion by the Co-ordination group and no referral to the CHMP/CVMP.(National Agencies will adopt the decision and will issue the marketing authorisation subject to submission of acceptable translations).

C. Numbering System for the Procedures for Mutual Recognition and Decentralised Procedure:

The numbering system is used for identification of procedures for mutual recognition. Each procedure is therefore characterised by a specific and unique number for unambiguous identification. The number for a specific procedure is a unique combination of six sections:

- CC/D/nnnn/sss/X/vvv
- C: the initials (2 digits) of the Reference Member State
- D: H for Human or V for Veterinary
- n: specific number (4 digits) for the actual medicinal product
- s: sequential speciality number. A separate number (3 digits) is allocated to each pharmaceutical form/strength and sequential numbering is used independent of whether the new presentation is a new pharmaceutical form or a new strength or a combination of both.
- X : Type of marketing application to the medicinal product :
    - "MR" for applications for marketing authorisation via MRP
    - "DC" for applications for marketing authorisation via DCP
    - "IA" for Type IA Notifications
    - "IB" for Type IB Notifications
    - "II" for Type II Variations

    - "R" for Renewals
    - "E" for Repeat-use Procedures
    - "O" for data bases when information in this section is not relevant

- v: sequential number (3 digits) for notifications/variations, renewals or repeat-use procedures. The sequential numbering is only applicable to a specific type of procedure (notifications/variations or renewals or repeat-use), thus creating three independent circles of sequential numbers.

D. Centralised authorisation procedure:

- Under the centralised authorisation procedure, pharmaceutical companies submit a single marketing-authorisation application to EMA. This allows the marketing-authorisation holder to market the medicine and make it available to patients and healthcare professionals throughout the EU on the basis of a single marketing authorisation. EMA's Committee for Medicinal products for Human Use (CHMP) or Committee for Medicinal products for Veterinary Use (CVMP) carry out a scientific assessment of the application and give a recommendation on whether the medicine should be marketed or not. Once granted by the European Commission the centralised marketing authorisation is valid in all EU Member States as well as in the European Economic Area (EEA) countries Iceland, Liechtenstein and Norway.

  The centralised procedure is **compulsory** for:

  i. Human medicines containing a new active substance to treat:

    - Human immunodeficiency virus (HIV) or acquired immune deficiency syndrome (AIDS).
    - Cancer.
    - Diabetes.
    - Neurodegenerative diseases.
    - Auto-immune and other immune dysfunctions.
    - Viral diseases.
    - Medicines derived from biotechnology processes, such as genetic engineering.

ii. Advanced-therapy medicines, such as gene-therapy, somatic cell-therapy or tissue-engineered medicines.

iii. Orphan medicines (medicines for rare diseases).

iv. Veterinary medicines for use as growth or yield enhancers.

It is **optional** for other medicines:

- containing new active substances for indications other than those stated above.
- that are a significant therapeutic, scientific or technical innovation.
- whose authorisation would be in the interest of public or animal health at EU level.

Today, **the great majority of new, innovative medicines** pass through the centralised authorisation procedure in order to be marketed in the EU.

a. **Flow Chart of the Centralised Procedure**

Centralised Procedure	
Day 1	Start the procedure for MAA
Day 70	Assessment Report from(co)-Rappoteur
Day 115	CHMP provides comments
Day 120	CHMP forwards to applicant list questions-Stop clock
Day 121	Submission of response by applicant
Day 150	Joint assessment report from (co)-Rappoteur
Day 170	Comments by CHMP
Day 180	CHMP Decision on need of oral explanation by applicant
Day 181	Oral explanation y applicant-Restart the clock
Day 185	Final Draft of English SPC, leaflets and labelling by applicant to co-rappoteur, EMEA,CHMP
Day 210	CHMP opinion

CHAPTER 27

Site Master File

Introduction

- Site Master file is self-explanatory notes to guide to the regulatory authority in planning and conducting GMP inspections for manufacturing site where all kind of manufacturing operations such as production, packaging and labelling, testing, relabeling and repackaging of all types of medicinal products are explained. A Site Master File should contain adequate information but, as far as possible not exceed 25-30 pages plus appendices. Simple plans outline drawings or schematic layouts are preferred instead of narratives. The Site Master File, including appendices, should be readable when printed on A4 paper sheets. The Site Master File should be a part of documentation belonging to the quality management system of the manufacturer and kept updated accordingly. The Site Master File should have an edition number, the date it becomes effective and the date by which it has to be reviewed. It should be subject to regular review to ensure that it is up to date and representative of current activities. Each Appendix can have an individual effective date, allowing for independent updating.

27.1 Content of Site Master File

A. GENERAL INFORMATION ON THE MANUFACTURER :

I. Contact information on the manufacturer

- Name and official address of the manufacturer.
- Names and street addresses of the site, buildings and production units located on the site.

- Contact information of the manufacturer including 24 hrs telephone number of the contact personnel in the case of product defects or recalls.
- Identification number of the site as e.g. GPS details, or any other geographic location system, D-U-N-S (Data Universal Numbering.
- System) Number (a unique identification number provided by Dun & Bradstreet) of the site 1.

II. Authorised pharmaceutical manufacturing activities of the site

- Copy of the valid manufacturing authorisation issued by the relevant Competent Authority in Appendix 1; or when applicable. If the Competent Authority does not issue manufacturing authorizations, this should be stated.
- Brief description of manufacture, import, export, distribution and other activities as authorized by the relevant competent authorities including foreign authorities with authorized dosage forms/activities, respectively; where not covered by the manufacturing authorization.
- Type of products currently manufactured on-site (list in Appendix 2) where not covered by Appendix 1.
- List of GMP inspections of the site within the last 5 years; including dates and name/country of the Competent Authority having performed the inspection. A copy of current GMP certificate (Appendix 3) should be included, if available.

III. Any other manufacturing activities carried out on the site

- Description of non-pharmaceutical activities on-site, if any.

B. QUALITY MANAGEMENT SYSTEM OF THE MANUFACTURER

I. The quality management system of the manufacturer

- Brief description of the quality management systems run by the company and reference to the standards used;

- Responsibilities related to the maintaining of quality system including senior management;
- Information of activities for which the site is accredited and certified, including dates and contents of accreditations, names of accrediting bodies.

II. Release procedure of finished products

- Detailed description of qualification requirements (education and work experience) of the Authorised Person(s)/Qualified Person(s) responsible for batch certification and releasing procedures;
- General description of batch certification and releasing procedure;
- Role of Authorised Person/Qualified Person in quarantine and release of finished products and in assessment of compliance with the Marketing Authorisation;
- The arrangements between Authorised Persons/ Qualified Persons when several Authorised Persons/ Qualified Persons are involved;
- Statement on whether the control strategy employs Process Analytical Technology (PAT) and/or Real Time Release or Parametric Release.

III. Management of suppliers and contractors

- A brief summary of the establishment/knowledge of supply chain and the external audit program.
- Brief description of the qualification system of contractors, manufacturers of active pharmaceutical ingredients (API) and other critical materials suppliers.
- Measures taken to ensure that products manufactured are compliant with TSE (Transmitting animal spongiform encephalopathy) guidelines.
- Measures adopted where counterfeit/falsified products, bulk products (i.e. unpacked tablets), active pharmaceutical ingredients or excipients are suspected or identified.
- Use of outside scientific, analytical or other technical assistance in relation to manufacture and analysis.

- List of contract manufacturers and laboratories including the addresses and contact information and flow charts of supply-chains for outsourced manufacturing and Quality Control activities; e.g. sterilization of primary packaging material for aseptic processes, testing of starting raw-materials etc, should be presented in Appendix 4.
- Brief overview of the responsibility sharing between the contract giver and acceptor with respect to compliance with the Marketing Authorization.

IV. Quality Risk Management (QRM)

- Brief description of QRM methodologies used by the manufacturer.
- Scope and focus of QRM including brief description of any activities which are performed at corporate level, and those which are performed locally. Any application of the QRM system to assess continuity of supply should be mentioned.

V. Product Quality Reviews

- Brief description of methodologies used.

C. PERSONNEL

- Organisation chart showing the arrangements for quality management, production and quality control positions/titles in Appendix 5, including senior management and Qualified Person(s).
- Number of employees engaged in the quality management, production, quality control, storage and distribution respectively.

D. PREMISES AND EQUIPMENT

a. Premises

- Short description of plant; size of the site and list of buildings. If the production for different markets, i.e. for local, EU, USA etc takes place in different buildings on the site, the buildings should be listed with destined markets identified.

- Simple plan or description of manufacturing areas with indication of scale (architectural or engineering drawings are not required).
- Lay outs and flow charts of the production areas (in Appendix 6) showing the room classification and pressure differentials between adjoining areas and indicating the production activities (i.e. compounding, filling, storage, packaging, etc.) in the rooms.
- Lay-outs of warehouses and storage areas, with special areas for the storage and handling of highly toxic, hazardous and sensitising materials indicated, if applicable.
- Brief description of specific storage conditions if applicable, but not indicated on the lay-outs.

I. Brief description of heating, ventilation and air conditioning (HVAC) systems

- Principles for defining the air supply, temperature, humidity, pressure differentials and air change rates, policy of air recirculation (%).

II. Brief description of water systems

- Quality references of water produced.
- Schematic drawings of the systems in Appendix 7.

III. Brief description of other relevant utilities, such as steam, compressed air, nitrogen, etc.

- Principles for defining the air supply, temperature, humidity, pressure differentials and air change rates, policy of air recirculation (%).

IV. Brief description of water systems

- Quality references of water produced.
- Schematic drawings of the systems in Appendix 7.

V. Brief description of other relevant utilities, such as steam, compressed air, nitrogen, etc.

a. Equipment:

- Listing of major production and control laboratory equipment with critical pieces of equipment identified should be provided in Appendix 8.

VI. Cleaning and sanitation

- Brief description of cleaning and sanitation methods of product contact surfaces (i.e. manual cleaning, automatic Clean-in-Place, etc).

VII. GMP critical computerised systems

- Description of GMP critical computerised systems (excluding equipment specific Programmable Logic Controllers (PLCs).

E. DOCUMENTATION

- Description of documentation system (i.e. electronic, manual).
- When documents and records are stored or archived off-site (including pharmacovigilance data, when applicable): List of types of documents/records; name and address of storage site and an estimate of time required retrieving documents from the off-site archive.

F. PRODUCTION

I. Type of products

(References to Appendix 1 or 2 can be made):

- Type of products manufactured including
  a. list of dosage forms of both human and veterinary products which are manufactured on the site.
  b. list of dosage forms of investigational medicinal products (IMP), manufactured for any clinical trials on the site, and when different from the commercial manufacturing, information of production areas and personnel.
- Toxic or hazardous substances handled (e.g. with high pharmacological activity and/or with sensitising properties).
- Product types manufactured in a dedicated facility or on a campaign basis, if applicable.
- Process Analytical Technology (PAT) applications, if applicable: general statement of the relevant technology, and associated computerized systems.

II. Process validation

- Brief description of general policy for process validation;
- Policy for reprocessing or reworking.

III. Material management and warehousing

- Arrangements for the handling of starting materials, packaging materials, bulk and finished products including sampling, quarantine, release and storage.
- Arrangements for the handling of rejected materials and products.

G. QUALITY CONTROL (QC)

- Description of the Quality Control activities carried out on the site in terms of physical, chemical, and microbiological and biological testing.

H. DISTRIBUTION, COMPLAINTS, PRODUCT DEFECTS AND RECALLS

I. Distribution (to the part under the responsibility of the manufacturer)

- Types (wholesale licence holders, manufacturing licence holders, etc) and locations (EU/EEA, USA, etc) of the companies to which the products are shipped from the site.
- Description of the system used to verify that each customer/recipient is legally entitled to receive medicinal products from the manufacturer.
- Brief description of the system to ensure appropriate environmental conditions during transit, e.g. temperature monitoring/control.
- Arrangements for product distribution and methods by which product traceability is maintained.
- Measures taken to prevent manufacturers' products to fall in the illegal supply chain.

II. Complaints, product defects and recalls

- Brief description of the system for handling complains, product defects and recalls.

I. SELF INSPECTIONS

- Short description of the self inspection system with focus on criteria used for selection of the areas to be covered during planned inspections, practical arrangements and follow-up activities.

27.2 Appendix

- Appendix 1 : Copy of valid manufacturing authorisation.
- Appendix 2 : List of dosage forms manufactured including the INN-names or common name (as available) of active pharmaceutical ingredients (API) used.
- Appendix 3 : Copy of valid GMP Certificate.
- Appendix 4 : List of contract manufacturers and laboratories including the addresses and contact information, and flow-charts of the supply chains for these outsourced activities.
- Appendix 5 : Organisational charts.
- Appendix 6 : Layouts of production areas including material and personnel flows, general flow charts of manufacturing processes of each product type (dosage form).
- Appendix 7 : Schematic drawings of water systems.
- Appendix 8 : List of major production and laboratory equipment.

CHAPTER 28

Standard Operating Procedure (SOP)

Introduction

- A Standard Operating Procedure (SOP) is a set of written instructions that document a routine or repetitive activity followed by an organization. The development and use of SOPs are an integral part of a successful quality system as it provides individuals with the information to perform a job properly, and facilitates consistency in the quality and integrity of a product or end-result. The term "SOP" may not always be appropriate and terms such as protocols, instructions, worksheets, and laboratory operating procedures may also be used. For this document "SOP" will be used. SOPs describe both technical and fundamental programmatic operational elements of an organization that would be managed under a work plan or a Quality Assurance (QA) Project Plan.
- SOPs detail the regularly recurring work processes that are to be conducted or followed within an organization. They document the way activities are to be performed to facilitate consistent conformance to technical and quality system requirements and to support data quality. They may describe, for example, fundamental programmatic actions and technical actions such as analytical processes, and processes for maintaining, calibrating, and using equipment. SOPs are intended to be specific to the organization or facility whose activities are described and assist that organization to maintain their quality control and quality assurance processes and ensure compliance with governmental regulations.

- If not written correctly, SOPs are of limited value. In addition, the best written SOPs will fail if they are not followed. Therefore, the use of SOPs needs to be reviewed and re-enforced by management, preferably the direct supervisor. Current copies of the SOPs also need to be readily accessible for reference in the work areas of those individuals actually performing the activity, either in hard copy or electronic format, otherwise SOPs serve little purpose.

28.1 Writing Styles

SOPs should be written in a concise, step-by-step, easy-to-read format. The information presented should be unambiguous and not overly complicated. The active voice and present verb tense should be used. The term "you" should not be used, but implied. The document should not be wordy, redundant, or overly lengthy. Keep it simple and short. Information should be conveyed clearly and explicitly to remove any doubt as to what is required. Also, use a flow chart to illustrate the process being described. In addition, follow the style guide used by your organization, e.g., font size and margins.

28.2 Sop Process

The organization should have a procedure in place for determining what procedures or processes need to be documented. Those SOPs should then be written by individuals knowledgeable with the activity and the organization's internal structure. These individuals are essentially subject-matter experts who actually perform the work or use the process. A team approach can be followed, especially for multi-tasked processes where the experiences of a number of individuals are critical, which also promotes "buy-in" from potential users of the SOP.

SOPs should be written with sufficient detail so that someone with limited experience with or knowledge of the procedure, but with a basic understanding, can successfully reproduce the procedure when unsupervised. The experience requirement for performing an activity should be noted in the section on personnel qualifications. For example, if a basic chemistry or biological course experience or additional training is required that requirement should be indicated.

28.3 SOP Review and Approval

SOPs should be reviewed (that is, validated) by one or more individuals with appropriate training and experience with the process. It is especially helpful if draft SOPs are actually tested by individuals other than the original writer before the SOPs are finalized.

The finalized SOPs should be approved as described in the organization's Quality Management Plan or its own SOP for preparation of SOPs. Generally the immediate supervisor, such as a section or branch chief, and the organization's quality assurance officer review and approve each SOP. Signature approval indicates that an SOP has been both reviewed and approved by management.

28.4 Frequency of Revisions and Reviews

SOPs need to remain current to be useful. Therefore, whenever procedures are changed, SOPs should be updated and re-approved. If desired, modify only the pertinent section of an SOP and indicate the change date/revision number for that section in the Table of Contents and the document control notation.

SOPs should be also systematically reviewed on a periodic basis, e.g. every 1-2 years, to ensure that the policies and procedures remain current and appropriate, or to determine whether the SOPs are even needed. The review date should be added to each SOP that has been reviewed. If an SOP describes a process that is no longer followed, it should be withdrawn from the current file and archived.

The review process should not be overly cumbersome to encourage timely review. The frequency of review should be indicated by management in the organization's Quality Management Plan. That plan should also indicate the individual(s) responsible for ensuring that SOPs are current.

Training should be provided (as necessary) when a document is revised or a new document is implemented.

28.5 Checklists

Many activities use checklists to ensure that steps are followed in order. Checklists are also used to document completed actions. Any checklists or forms included as part of an activity should be referenced at the points in the procedure where they are to be used and then attached to the SOP.

In some cases, detailed checklists are prepared specifically for a given activity. In those cases, the SOP should describe, at least generally, how the checklist is to be prepared, or on what it is to be based. Copies of specific checklists should be then maintained in the file with the activity results and/or with the SOP.

Remember that the checklist is not the SOP, but a part of the SOP.

28.6 Document Control

Each organization should develop a numbering system to systematically identify and label their SOPs, and the document control should be described in its Quality Management Plan. Generally, each page of an SOP should have control documentation notation, similar to that illustrated below. A short title and identification (ID) number can serve as a reference designation. The revision number and date are very useful in identifying the SOP in use when reviewing historical data and is critical when the need for evidentiary records is involved and when the activity is being reviewed. When the number of pages is indicated, the user can quickly check if the SOP is complete. Generally this type of document control notation is located in the upper right-hand corner of each document page following the title page.

Short Title/ID # Rev. #: Date: Page 1 of

28.7 SOP Document Tracking and Archival

The organization should maintain a master list of all SOPs. This file or database should indicate the SOP number, version number, date of issuance, title, author, status, organizational division, branch, section, and any historical information regarding past versions. The QA Manager (or designee) is generally the individual responsible for maintaining a file listing all current quality-related SOPs used within the organization. If an electronic database is used, automatic "Review SOP" notices can be sent. Note that this list may be used also when audits are being considered or when questions are raised as to practices being followed within the organization.

The Quality Management Plan should indicate the individual(s) responsible for assuring that only the current version is used. That plan should also designated where, and how, outdated versions are to be maintained or archived in a manner to prevent their continued use, as well as to be available for historical data review.

Electronic storage and retrieval mechanisms are usually easier to access than a hard-copy document format. For the user, electronic access can be limited to a read-only format, thereby protecting against unauthorized changes made to the document.

28.8 SOP General Format

SOPs should be organized to ensure ease and efficiency in use and to be specific to the organization which develops it. There is no one "correct" format; and internal formatting will vary with each organization and with the type of SOP being written. Where possible break the information into a series of logical steps to avoid a long list. The level of detail provided in the SOP may differ based on, e.g., whether the process is critical, the frequency of that procedure being followed, the number of people who will use the SOP, and where training is not routinely available. A generalized format is discussed next.

I. Title Page

The first page or cover page of each SOP should contain the following information: a title that clearly identifies the activity or procedure, an SOP identification (ID) number, date of issue and/or revision, the name of the applicable agency, division, and/or branch to which this SOP applies, and the signatures and signature dates of those individuals who prepared and approved the SOP. Electronic signatures are acceptable for SOPs maintained on a computerized database.

II. Table of Contents

A Table of Contents may be needed for quick reference, especially if the SOP is long, for locating information and to denote changes or revisions made only to certain sections of an SOP.

III. Text

- Well-written SOPs should first briefly describe the purpose of the work or process, including any regulatory information or standards that are appropriate to the SOP process, and the scope to indicate what is covered. Define any specialized or unusual terms either in a separate definition section or in the appropriate discussion section. Denote what sequential procedures should be followed, divided into significant sections; e.g., possible interferences, equipment needed, personnel qualifications, and safety considerations (preferably listed in bold to capture the attention of the user). Finally, describe next all appropriate QA and quality control (QC) activities for that procedure, and list any cited or significant references.

- As noted above, SOPs should be clearly worded so as to be readily understandable by a person knowledgeable with the general concept of the procedure, and the procedures should be written in a format that clearly describes the steps in order. Use of diagrams and flow charts help to break up long sections of text and to briefly summarize a series of steps for the reader.
- Attach any appropriate information, e.g., an SOP may reference other SOPs. In such a case, the following should be included:

    a. Cite the other SOP and attach a copy, or reference where it may be easily located.

    b. If the referenced SOP is not to be followed exactly, the required modification should be specified in the SOP at the section where the other SOP is cited.

<table>
<tr><th colspan="4">STANDARD OPERATION PROCEDURE</th></tr>
<tr><td colspan="4">Title</td></tr>
<tr><td>SOP No. and Version No</td><td></td><td>Department</td><td></td></tr>
<tr><td>Effective Date</td><td></td><td>Page No</td><td></td></tr>
<tr><td colspan="4"></td></tr>
<tr><td colspan="4">1. Objective
2. Scope
3. Responsibility
4. Definition
5. To be Reviewed Before
6. Procedure
7. Reference
8. Abbreviations
9. Annexure
10. Format</td></tr>
<tr><td>Prepared By
(Sign and Date)</td><td colspan="2">Reviewed By
(Sign and Date)</td><td>Approved By
(Sign and Date)</td></tr>
</table>

28.9 Definitions

i. **Appendix:** An appendix is a section added at the end of a document to provide additional information.

ii. **Controlled Copy:** A formal copy of the latest, approved version of a document. A controlled copy must be systematically tracked, updated and stored for use.

iii. **Uncontrolled Copy:** An informal copy of a document for which no attempt is made to update it after distribution. Copies of documents made by users (in paper or electronic form) are considered "uncontrolled copies". The responsibility of making sure a document is the most current approved document is with the user of the document. Documented Information: information required to be controlled and maintained by an organization and the medium on which it is contained. (ISO 9000:2015(E))

iv. **Effectiveness:** Extent to which planned activities are realized and planned results achieved. (ISO 9000:2015 (E))

v. **Effective Date:** Date the documents are signed by the Chair person and it officially begins to be used.

vi. **Form:** A document used to facilitate procedural implementation or document procedural objectives.

vii. **Document Control**: Ensuring that documents are reviewed for adequacy, approved for release, distributed to and used at the location where the prescribed activity is performed. Obsolete documents are to be retained.

<table>
<tr><th colspan="10">Document Issue, Retrieval and Reconciliation Register</th></tr>
<tr><td colspan="10">Document Name :</td></tr>
<tr><td colspan="6">Issuance Detail</td><td colspan="4">Retrieval Details</td></tr>
<tr><td>Date of issuance</td><td>Document no/Format no/Checklist No</td><td>No.Copy issued</td><td>Receiving Department</td><td>Issued By (Sign and Date)</td><td>Issued to (Sign and Date)</td><td>Return By (Sign and Date)</td><td>Received By (Sign and Date)</td><td>Destroyed By (Sign and Date</td><td>Remark</td></tr>
<tr><td></td><td></td><td></td><td></td><td></td><td></td><td></td><td></td><td></td><td></td></tr>
</table>

viii. **Document Number:** A unique identifier assigned by the firm to differentiate documents (Procedure, Form or Guidance) and their versions. All document numbers will include a standard prefix and a unique alpha-numeric identifier for a type of document and its version.

ix. **Form Number:** A unique alpha-numeric identifier assigned by the firm used to differentiate forms and their versions. The

Form Number consists of a prefix "F" (Form) followed by five digits. The first four digits designate the procedure the form is associated with. The next digit indicates the sequential number of the form.

x. **Implementation Date:** Date that staff has received training and documents are posted to use.

xi. **Master Document List:** A list of released documents maintained by the firm and including the Document Number, Version date, Revision Date and Publication Date.

xii. **Master file:** This file includes all signed original documents and all electronic files.

xiii. **Document History Record:** The Document History Record contains version and publication dates, document and version numbers, approval signatures, and revision records.

Document History Record			
SOP Name and Number	**Version No and Effective date**	**Description of changes**	**Changes done by**

CHAPTER 29

Quality Manual

Introduction

The quality manual is a document that a facility writes to explain which portions of which regulations are applicable to the facility and which documents the policies, procedures, responsibilities, and documentation, that must be in place for the facility to comply with these regulatory responsibilities

A quality manual is required for implementing a quality management system. Such a system aims primarily at achieving customer satisfaction by meeting customer requirements through application of the system, continuous improvement of the system, and prevention of the occurrence of nonconformities.

The organization should establish and maintain a quality manual that includes

- The quality policy.
- The scope of the quality management system, including details of and justification for any exclusions.
- The documented procedures established for the quality management system, or reference to them, and
- A description of the interaction between the processes of the quality management system.

I. Contents of the Quality Manual

- A quality manual is a document that a facility writes to explain which regulations are applicable to the facility (i.e. which regulations will be followed by the facility.)
- The regulations that are to be followed are based on the process(es) that are performed at the facility.

- The facility's Quality Manual should outline which regulations are going to be followed, how they are going to be followed, who is responsible for ensuring that the regulations are followed, and which of the companies approved procedures address the regulations to be followed. If all parts of a regulation are not going to be followed, a facility may want to include a brief explanation as to why a part of a regulation is not applicable to the facility and therefore will not be outlined in the Quality Manual.
- The Quality Manual should be written in general terms with minimal specifics. The format of a Quality Manual is usually different than the format used for the facility's other approved documents. The format should still include such things as a facility's name, version control, and approval signatures.

  a. **Table of Contents:** A list of the sections contained within the Quality Manuel and the page each section begins on.

  b. **Introduction:** A brief description of the facility, the facility's purpose for writing a Quality Manual, and a brief description of the scope of the Quality Manual.

  c. **Facility Background:** List the name of the facility, where the facility is located, what radiopharmaceutical products are produced at the facility, and how these will be distributed.

  d. **Purpose:** Provide general statements explaining why and how the Quality Manual will be used.

  e. **Scope:** List the regulations that will be followed by the facility as well as any portions of the regulations that will not be followed. Provide a justification for why those portions of the regulations are not going to be followed.

  f. **Quality Policies and Objectives:** Include a brief statement about the approach that the facility is taking in regards to quality, (i.e. a Quality Mission Statement) and list the quality objectives of the facility. The quality objectives should not be numerous (five to seven is a typical number) and should be briefly stated.

  g. **Organization and Structure of Documentation:** Provide an explanation as to how the documentation structure at your facility is organized and managed in relation to the applicable regulations.

h. **Products:** This section should include a brief description of the products that are made and distributed by the facility including what the intended use of the products is to be. This description should be similar to a marketing type summary in that it does not list proprietary or explicit product information that would be detrimental to the facility if persons outside the facility read the description. This section should provide enough detail to justify the sections of the regulations that are and are not going to be followed.

i. **References:** A list of all the different regulations that were sited within the Quality Manual.

j. **Quality Policies for Specific Regulation Elements:** This section will encompass the majority of the manual. It will include each regulation that will be followed by the facility, a brief description of how the facility intends to follow the regulation, and a list of the approved documents (by document name and number) that the facility has in place which specifically address/discuss the facility's policies and objectives as stated in this section of the Quality Manual.

II. Topics that should be covered in the final section on Quality Policies for Specific Regulation Elements

A. Quality Systems

The Quality System ensures that the product complies with its specified requirements and is manufactured in accordance with appropriate standards.

The Quality System is documented on four levels:

a. Level 1 Quality Policy

b. Level 2 Quality Manual

c. Level 3 Standard Operating Procedures

d. Level 4 Quality Records and Logbooks

B. Deviations and Events

- Event Recording
- Reviews and Investigations
- Remediation

C. Change Control

- Change Initiation and Approval
- Change Execution and Tracking
- Change Verification and Closure

D. Audit Management

- Planning
- Execution
- Review and Remediation

E. Document Management

- Storing and Classification
- Access and Viewing
- Creating New Documents
- Lifecycle Managements
- Printing

F. Training Management

- Employee Course Management
- Training Request and Approval
- Gap Management and Records

G. Equipment Management

- Inventory Management
- Preventative Maintenance
- Remedial Maintenance

H. General Requirements

- Security and Access Control
- Facility Management
- Corrective Action Preventive Action (CAPA)
- CAPA Initiation
- Investigations and Action Plan
- CAPA Closure

I. Validation

- Documentation Structure and Formats
- Change Control
- Planning and Scheduling
- Roles and Responsibilities
- Regulatory Requirements for Testing

J. A list of SOPs, Forms, Validation Documentation and other appendicies

K. Format

<table>
<tr><th colspan="3">QUALITY MANUAL</th></tr>
<tr><td colspan="2">Function: Quality Assurance Department</td><td>Effective Date:</td></tr>
<tr><td colspan="2">Document: Quality Manrual</td><td>Version: 01</td></tr>
<tr><td colspan="2">Next Review Date:</td><td></td></tr>
<tr><td>Prepared by:
Sign and Date</td><td>Reviewed by:
Sign and Date</td><td>Approved by:
Sign and Date</td></tr>
</table>

L. Contents

SECTION AND TITLE	PAGE
1. Introduction 2. Organization 3. Manufacturing Facility 4. Quality System 5. Management Responsibility 6. Design and Change Control 7. Document Control 8. Purchasing and Vendor Assurance 9. Material and Product Identification and Traceability 10. Process Control Programmes 11. Inspection and Testing Programmes 12. Calibration Programmes 13. Inspection and Test Status 14. Control of Non-Conforming Product 15. Corrective and Preventive Action Systems 16. Handling and Storage of Materials and Products 17. Control of Quality Records 18. Internal Quality Audits 19. Training Programmes 20. Statistical Techniques 21. Computer Systems Management 22. Facility Control 23. Management of Equipment and Critical Process Utilities 24. Validation Programmes 25. Risk Assessment 26. Occupational Safety and Health Programmes	

CHAPTER 30

Human Error Reduction: Pharma Industry Challenge

Introduction

Pharmaceutical companies often cite human error as the sole cause of a noncompliance issue. In Pharmaceutical industry, identifying and reducing the occurrence of human is not always so rigorously assessed during investigations. Common corrective actions for human error within a GMP production facility often include retraining or awareness sessions combined with document updates or revisions that include additional document checks and signatures. In most cases, no scientific rationale for human error as root cause. Investigation corrective actions focused on retraining, typically do not fix the true root cause and generally will not prevent a reoccurrence of the issue. Simply retraining using existing protocols is unlikely to address the recurring errors. If staff have been trained on the current versions of the procedures, it is difficult to justify, in many cases, why retraining should be included as a preventative action. This chapter discuss about how Regulatory and industry see the human error, human error reduction, power of 5-WHY, techniques for strong CAPAs, Root cause analyses and cGMP improvements.

Human behavior is complex and just like equipment, product, and process it needs to be analyzed in depth. Take the example of day to day, Chemical engineers explain product behavior, mechanical engineers explain equipment behavior, industrial engineers explain process behavior, but who explains human behavior? The reality is that people make mistakes because systems allows. The problem basically relies in the fact that most of the systems do not directly consider human error prevention as part of the design and human factors and capabilities are usually ignored when it comes to people.

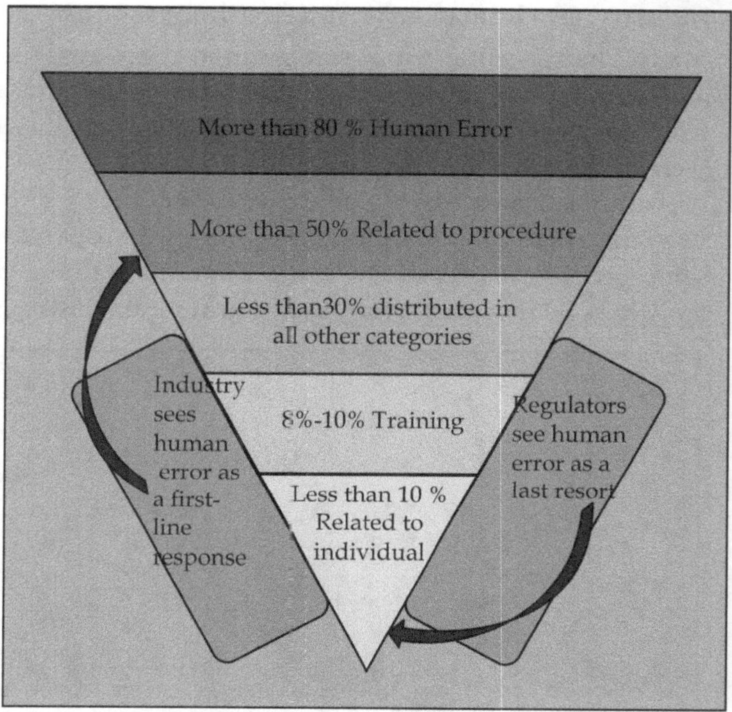

30.1 How do Industry and Regulatory Expectations and Approaches Differ?

A. **Regulators** see human error as a last resort Figure-1

Expectation is that you can - *and have* - eliminated any possible process issues and confirmed that the individual had everything they needed and simply wasn't focused.

- Regulatory expectation are moving towards a science- and risk-based.
- Approach to develop and document scientific rationales for classifying and preventing human error.
- Integrating human error reduction tools within a quality system.
- Need not be cumbersome or complicated. Pharmaceutical companies can utilize the Talsico human error reduction methodology, to categorize human error and also to develop effective strategies for prevention.

B. Industry sees human error as a first-line response

Many Pharmaceutical industry assume processes, procedures and training are bulletproof, and the issue *must* have resulted from someone not paying appropriate attention to what they were doing at the time. When we do look at our training, procedures or process, we often verify that they make sense to *us* - the reviewer. And then we retrain the operator on the same process or procedure, using the same training process - *quickly!* - So they can return to performing the task again.

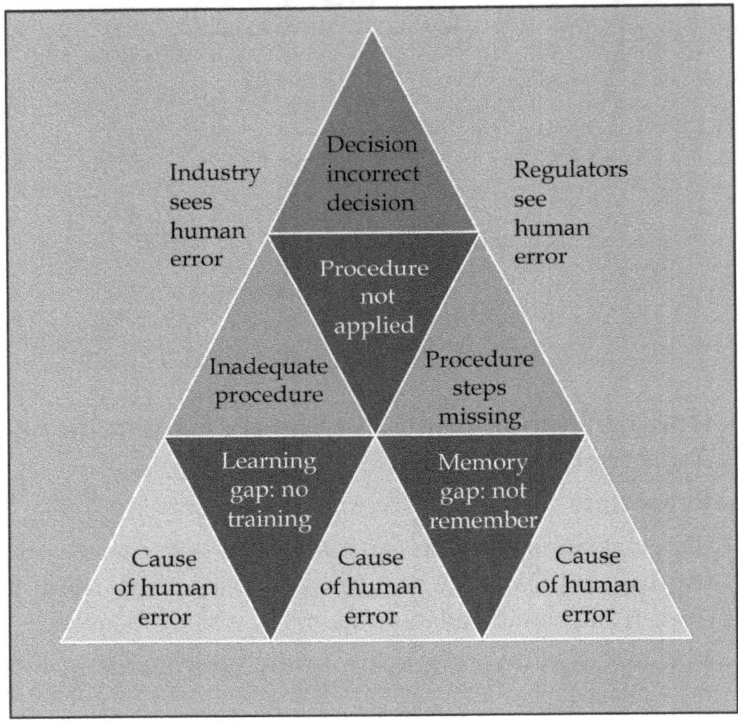

30.2 Understanding, Investigation & Tackling of human Error

- *First Aim*: For any given problem, workflow assures that the right people, have the right information, at the right time.
- When tackling the persistent problem of quality failures deemed to be caused by human error it is important to begin with a basic understanding of its structure and root cause with corrective and preventive action.

30.3 Power of 5-WHY

5-Why root cause analysis method is simple in concept but requires real evidence, sure logic and great discipline in its use to find the true root cause of a failure event, investigation or problem by method of questioning to the identification of root cause(s) of a problem. 5 Why can be made effective by Involvement of the right people, avoid blaming - look for systemic problems and get creative. Through asking "Why?" repeatedly, you begin to understand what led to the problem - and ultimately identify the root cause. A "5 Whys" analysis can help you meet the regulatory expectation of assessing whether process, procedure, or system based problems contributed to a human error. If we go through the analysis and find nothing but the operator making an honest error, you can be confident in - and able to support - your assessment of human error as the root cause.

30.4 Human Error and Retraining

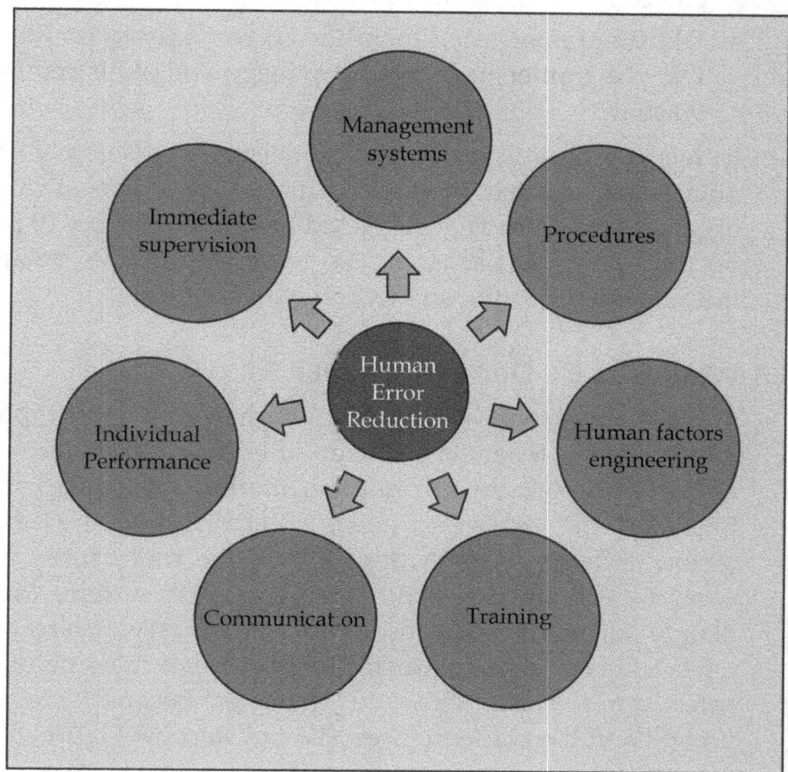

- Training is usually used as a corrective action for human error. Although training has proven to be effective for transferring knowledge, skills and abilities (KSA's), it will only work for new employees, new processes or to instruct on changes to existing processes if the employees that will perform the task lack the new KSA's. Prior to calling CAPA as training for a human error following questions can ask for training program:
    a. Did the training reflect the procedure content and are all operators performing the task doing it the same way?
    b. Was it the operator's first time performing the task independently? Were they allowed enough practice on the task, or was training rushed? Was training time used for appropriate training activities?
    c. Did the trainer verify the operator's ability to perform each required element of the task? Against what standard?
    d. Is all the information the trainee needs to perform the task correctly accessible to them?
    e. Did the trainer teach them the correct way to do the task? Did the trainer have the knowledge and skills required to teach it?
- In fact, training is responsible for less that 10 percent of the deviations related to performance, yet most of the organization's efforts are directed towards less than 10 percent of the actual weaknesses. No wonder CAPA's related to training end up being so ineffective.

30.5 What Can Be Done for Human Error?

- The most effective way to control human error is to implement good systems. Systems take care of human factors (any aspect of the workplace or job implementation that makes it more likely for the worker to make an error) as well as external factors. Effective CAPA depends on the root cause and just want to elimate that root cause from the system. Motivate people to do things right when no one is watching, things need to make sense to them. People break rules because the rules don't make sense to them or because they don't understand the consequences. We can start by: Figure -3.

30.6 Measure of Human Error

- Human error can be prevented. Good and accurate administrative management systems which assure that there are controls for providing clear, accurate procedures, instructions and other aids are crucial for human error prevention. In addition, good human factors engineering of control systems, appropriate processes and work environment; job-relevant training and practice; appropriate supervision; good communications; and individual personnel performance, are all part of the formula human error prevention. Humans have more things in common than differences and after visiting many places in the world we can say that the areas requiring improvement are practically universal. We as humans don't operate in a vacuum. Behaviors are influenced by external as well as internal variables. Individuals are certainly responsible for their actions. But before we determine that internal factors like attitude or attention are responsible for the mistake, we as organizations are responsible for eliminating the possibilities of external factor influencing human behavior. Individual performance in manufacturing is proven to be responsible for less than five percent of deviations. And people want to do things right.

CHAPTER 31

Regulatory Inspections: Face Challenges through Proactive Measures

Introduction

Changes in regulatory audit focus, introduction stringent focus on compliance in pharmaceutical sector. Globally, Pharma organizations shall have to embrace a holistic approach. This involves aligning complex and disparate risks and regulatory compliance activities to the overall corporate strategy. The approach should be structured and incorporate a well-designed reporting and monitoring mechanism to provide a reasonable degree of assurance to management, boards, and audit committees. To be effective regulatory expectation, organizations must adhere all the elements and shall have central idea of the holistic approach to compliance management, which helps in the understanding compliance and continuous process. This chapter discuss about regulatory expectations, MEQVR -IPO Model, Pillar of compliance, Audit Trail Assessments and An Approach to Managing Regulatory Risks and Achieving Compliance

31.1 Regulatory Expectations?

- A robust system for the continuous improvements necessary to assure the safety, identity, strength, quality, and purity of drug products.
- CGMP in practices for 24hrs
- Linking Product, Process and Patient
- Adopting QbD design
- Quality Culture

- Quality System Elements
- Statistical Process Controls
- Continuous improvements

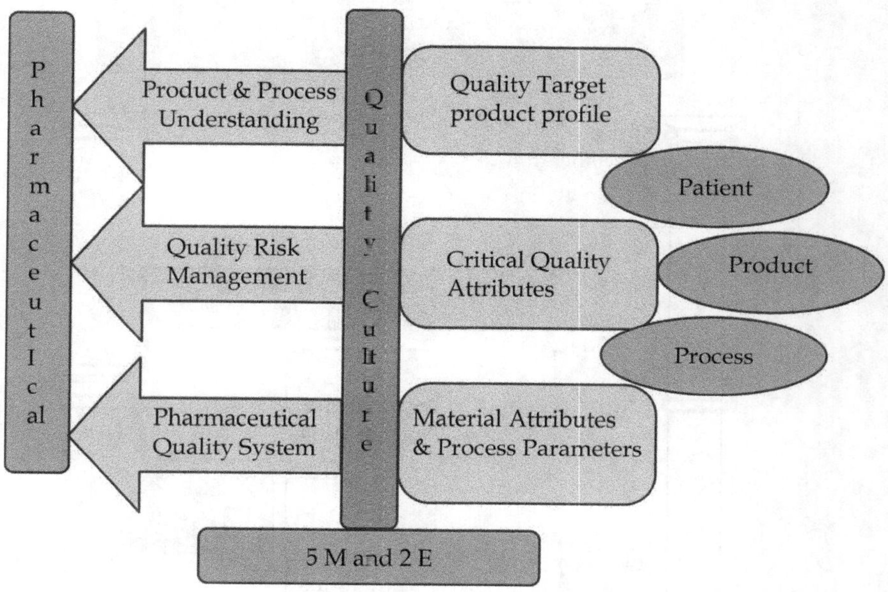

31.2 Current Regulatory Audits Looking

- Data integrity
- GxP Systems and Controls
- Chromatographic issues
- Risk Assessment
- Investigation
- Documentation Control
- GAP analysis
- Paper work sheet
- Security controls
- Audit Trails
- CAPA effectiveness
- Training

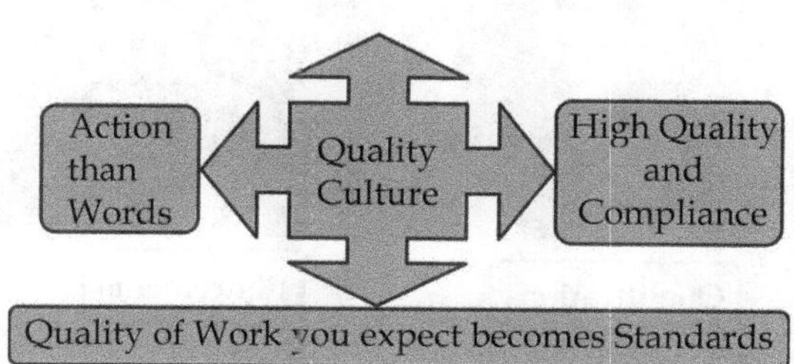

31.3 Regulators Looks at ....

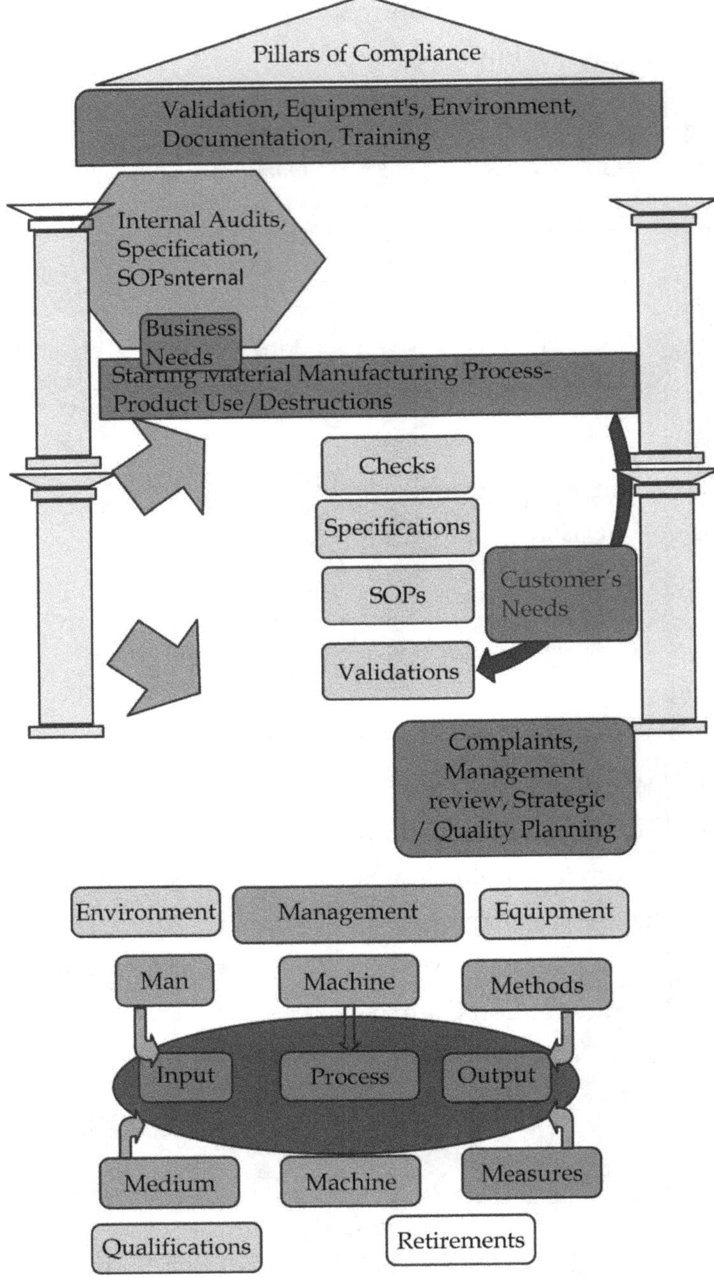

MEQVR –IPO Model

- Regulators are looking every pillars of compliance from process design, process Qualification and continuous process verification. Pillars of Compliance mainly depends on 7 M, 2 E, 1 Q, 1 V and 1 R which will be through Strong QMS system.
- **Risk-based approach:** Conduct appropriate levels of GxP impact and criticality risk assessment of systems and system functionality early in the planning stage and then throughout the validation life cycle as required.
- **Computer System Validation:** Map the stages and terminology of "Information systems", e.g., enterprise resource planning (ERP) and Laboratory Information Management Systems (LIMS) with the recognized validation life cycle model.
- **Cleaning Validation:** Appropriate and sensitive method to determine low level to meet MACO.

31.4 Audit Trail Assessments

The audit trail assessment is the first and the most critical steps to implement audit trail reviews. An inventory of all impacted systems need to be created to identify whether each individual system provide audit trails that are adequate and that can be used for performing the reviews. System level risk assessments need to be performed to identify whether the system is high, medium or low risk. The system risk needs to be used to prioritize the audit trail assessment and implementation of periodic reviews. Once the audit trail assessment are performed, system risk identified and all corrective actions are closed the audit trail reviews can be implemented. Prior to implementation the impact to resource need to be well understood based on the expected volume of work. Once this impact is understood hiring and reassigning of resource need to be completed prior to formal implementation.

Each functional area that have GxP computer systems need to perform the audit trail assessment to determine the following:

- Who has access to view the audit trails?
- Can the audit trail be printed from the application?
- Can the reviewer select a data range?
- Can the reviewer select a specific activity of interest during the audit trail review?

- Will it feasible to include the audit trail with the data results?
- Will it be feasible for QC systems to include the audit trail with the assay results?
- Are user's action time and date stamped?
- Does the audit trail records creation, modification and deletion of records?

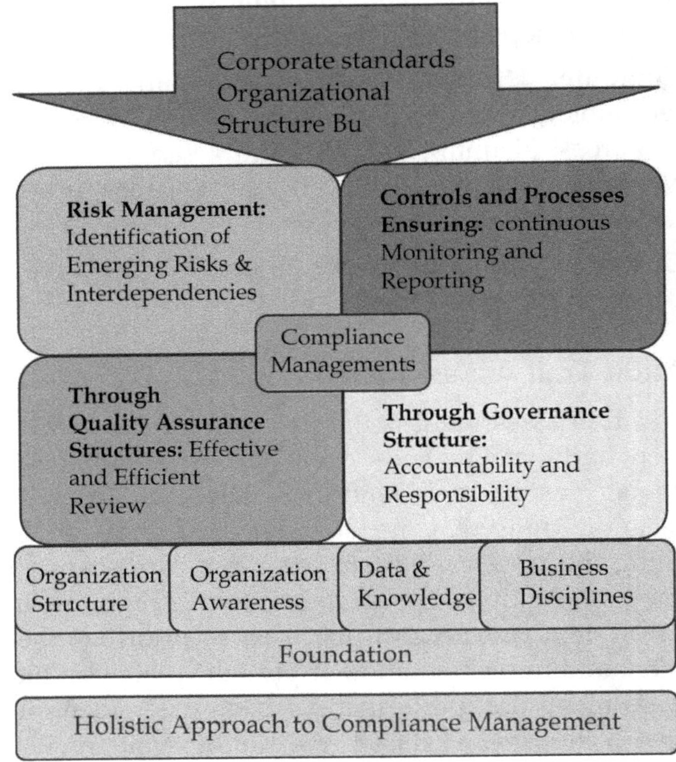

31.5 An Approach to Managing Regulatory Risks and Achieving Compliance

- Effective compliance management integrates risk management, controls and processes, and assurance and governance structures using tools and data. This should be backed by a strong organizational culture, an enterprise-wide awareness program, and business discipline. This holistic approach to the management of compliance will lead to greater awareness of regulation and help with the implementation of a focused plan to mitigate non-compliance and continuous process and not a one-time project.

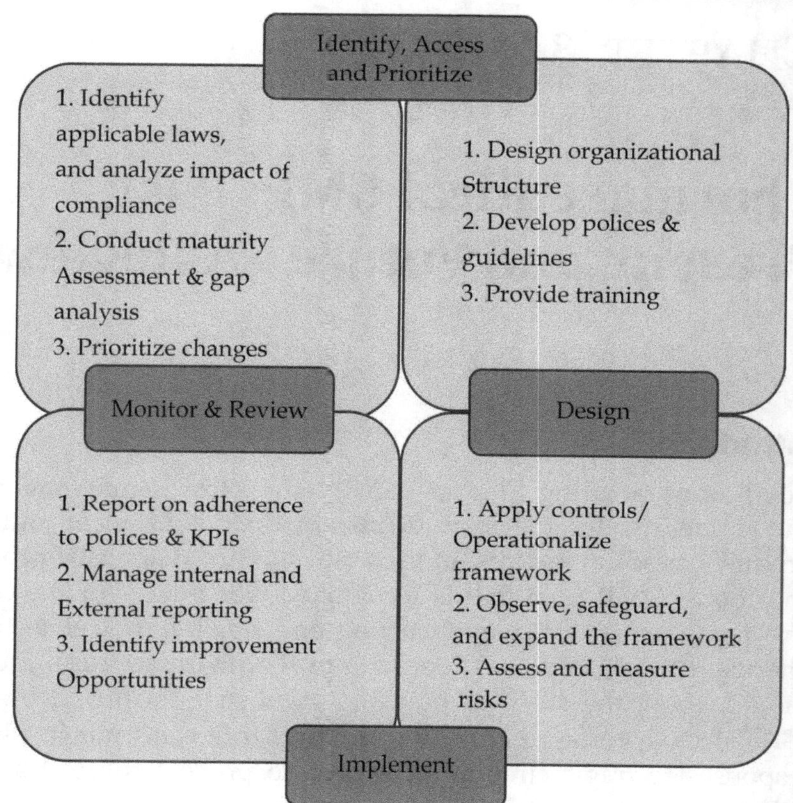

31.6 Measures of Regulatory Inspections

- When looking at the industry from a global standpoint it is clear that there are opportunities to address un-met regulatory requirements. Organized structure, awareness, knowledge management, policy, standards play an important roles in regulatory compliance environment. Due very complex industry, making the changes necessary will not be easy, and it will not happen overnight. To be successful in the future, we have to find ways to meets regulatory requirements today and the future by awareness, training, scientific and technology work with all stakeholders. As companies embark on this journey, we need to devote as much time and effort to clearly communicate the strategies to employees, customers and other stakeholders, planning for change and structuring their organizations for success.

CHAPTER 32

Pharmaceutical GMP: Past, Present, and Future - A Review

Introduction

Good Manufacturing Practice (GMP) is a set of regulations, codes, and guidelines for the manufacture of drug substances and drug products, medical devices, in vivo and in vitro diagnostic products, and foods. GMP term that is recognized worldwide for the control and management of manufacturing and quality control testing of pharmaceutical products. Everyone in the pharmaceutical industry should know the story of how the good manufacturing practices (GMPs) have come to be. Most requirements were put in place as responses to tragic circumstances and to prevent future tragedies. To obtain and maintain GMP compliance, one should know the precedent of the GMP. The present review highlights past, present and future of GMP .A GMP is a system for ensuring that products are consistently produced and controlled according to quality standards. It is designed to minimize the risks involved in any pharmaceutical production that cannot be eliminated through testing the final product. GMP covers all aspects of production from the starting materials, premises and equipment to the training and personal hygiene of staff. Detailed, written procedures are essential for each process that could affect the quality of the finished product. There must be systems to provide documented proof that correct procedures are consistently followed at each step in the manufacturing process - every time a product is made.

32.1 Current Expectations for Pharmaceutical Quality Systems

- Lifecycle Quality Risk Management : Addressing Two Major "Common Causes" of Variation.

- A Quality Culture that leads to Sustainable Compliance.
- Inspections of the Pharmaceutical Quality System.
- cGMP-compliant Quality System.
- Risk Reduction Opportunities Deficient Facilities and Processes.
- Open vs. Closed Processes (Also, Unit Operations vs. Integrated).
- Manually Intensive Operations vs. Automation.
- Human Error still very prominent root cause...
- Human Error is cause of substantial variation across the industry.
- Can be prevented by analyzing process for failure modes and increasing automation. A lifecycle QRM opportunity... "Human Error Analysis" – HE training allows for "deeper.

32.2 A Quality Culture That Leads to Sustainable Compliance

Leadership and the Corporate Quality Culture

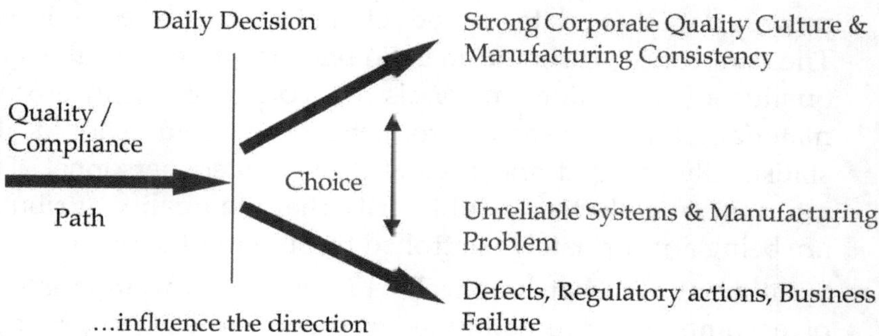

32.3 Quality Culture

- Support for the Quality Organization
- Actions More than Words
- Investment in Quality
- Quality Involved in Business Decision
- The Quality of the work you accept become your standard
- Organizational Structure: Assurance that QA is independent and not subordinate to the other organizational unit

32.4 Building Knowledge, Effective Monitoring & Control Systems

- To develop and use effective monitoring and control systems for process performance and product quality, thereby providing assurance of continued suitability and capability of processes."
- Control Procedures (monitor the output and validate the performance of manufacturing processes).
- Investigation of Discrepancies (Any unexplained discrepancy shall be thoroughly investigated. A written record of the investigation shall be made and shall include the conclusions and follow up.)
- Quality Unit Responsibilities (complete investigation of errors that have occurred).
- For each drug, evaluate the quality standards of each drug product to determine the need for changes in drug product specifications or manufacturing or control procedures at least annually.
- An ongoing program to collect and analyze product and process data that relate to product quality must be established. The data collected should include relevant process trends and quality of incoming materials or components, in-process material, and finished products. The data should be statistically trended and reviewed by trained personnel. The information collected should verify that the quality attributes are being appropriately controlled throughout the process.
- Scrutiny of intra-batch as well as inter-batch variation is part of a comprehensive continued process verification program (lifecycle stage 3).
- Ensure a timely and effective communication and escalation process exists to raise quality issues to the appropriate levels of management.

32.5 Global Supply Chain and Vendor Qualification

Vendor qualification program should provide adequate evidence that the manufacturer can consistently provide reliable and safe materials. Suppliers should be monitored and regularly scrutinized to assure ongoing reliability. It is your responsibility to ensure that raw materials received are suitable and approved by the quality unit prior to use.

32.6 Bundling GMP Enforcement with Other Violations

- FDA appears to have become more aggressive in its use of GMP Warning Letters to notify drug companies about violative conduct in other areas of their business. In some cases, the FDA has alerted companies that some of their products lack the necessary FDA approvals. In others, the agency has raised concerns about a company's promotional activities. In still other cases, the FDA has notified companies that they are violating FDA's pharmacy compounding rules.
- We fully expect this trend to continue in the future. As the agency continues to face an increasingly large number of enforcement priorities with limited resources, we believe that this "bundling" approach to enforcement will become more common. In addition to the areas of enforcement listed above, we think it is extremely likely that the FDA will focus on pharmacovigilance systems and adverse event reporting during future GMP inspections. This is especially true in light of the agency's heightened sensitivity to drug safety.

32.7 Quality Systems

The following quotations from recent Warning Letters illustrate FDA's concern in this area:

- [The observed GMP deficiencies are] indicative of your quality control unit not fulfilling its responsibility to assure the identity, strength, quality and purity of your manufactured product.
- Please explain why your firm's Quality Control Unit (QCU) did not detect and document these deficiencies during their batch production and control and what actions will be taken to assure these deficiencies do not extend to other batches of the same or other drug product.
- Failure to conduct investigations in a timely manner and to extend the investigations to other drug products that may have been impacted by the same failure while investigations of confirmed cross-contamination (without a probable root cause identified) were ongoing demonstrate the failure of your QCU to provide adequate oversight and ensure procedures are followed.

- These passages underscore the critical role that Quality Control Units play in pharmaceutical manufacturing and how closely the FDA monitors their performance.

32.8 Change Control: New FDA Expectations for Equipment Changes

The U.S. Food and Drug Administration (FDA) has published a new Manufacturing Equipment Addendum for the SUPAC Guidelines (Scale-up and post-approval changes), describing the administration's expectations when assessing manufacturing equipment changes.

This Guidance for Industry combines and supersedes the following Guidances:

- SUPAC-IR/MR: Immediate Release and Modified Release Solid Oral Dosage Forms, Manufacturing Equipment Addendum.
- SUPAC-SS: Nonsterile Semisolid Dosage Forms, Manufacturing Equipment Addendum.
- The biggest alteration was the removal of the lists of specific manufacturing equipment that were in both guidance. It now contains general information on SUPAC equipment. The reason is that FDA was concerned that misinterpretation of the lists could discourage advancements in manufacturing technologies.

  Furthermore, it clarifies the types of processes being referenced. The information in the document is presented in broad categories of unit operation. For each operation, equipment is categorized by class (operating principle) and subclass (design characteristic). Examples of types of equipment, but not specific brand information, are now given within the subclasses.

  When assessing manufacturing equipment changes; FDA recommends to follow "a risk-based approach that includes a rationale and complies with the regulations, including the cGMP regulations". They also recommend "addressing the impact on the product quality attributes of equipment variations (via process parameters) when designing and developing the manufacturing process".

References

1. Australian GMP Guidelines
    - Questions & answers on the code of good manufacturing practice for medicinal products.
    - Technical Guidance on the Interpretation of Manufacturing Standards for Supplier Qualification.
2. Canadian GMP Guidelines
    - Annex 2 to the Current Edition of the Good Manufacturing Practices Guidelines Schedule D Drugs (Biological Drugs) (GUI-0027).
    - Consultation: Draft Documents for Drug Good Manufacturing Practices Inspection Program (7 August 2009).
        - Consultation on Good Manufacturing Practices-Inspection Program Review (26 January 2011).
        - Drug Good Manufacturing Practices (GMP) and Establishment Licensing (EL) Enforcement Directive (POL-0004).
        - GMP Inspection Policy for Canadian Drug Establishments (POL-0011).
        - Good Manufacturing Practices - Audit Report Form (FRM-0211).
        - Good Manufacturing Practices - Audit Report Form (FRM-0211) Instructions.
        - Good Manufacturing Practices - Foreign Site Submission Form (FRM-0212).
        - Good Manufacturing Practices - Request for an Inspection of a Foreign Site Form (FRM-0213).
        - Good Manufacturing Practices - Foreign Site Inspection Services Agreement Form (FRM-0214).

- Good Manufacturing Practices (GMP) for Schedule D Drugs, Part 2, Human Blood and Blood Components.
- Good Manufacturing Practices (GMP) Guidelines (4 March 2011).
- Guidance Document - Annex 13 to the Current Edition of the Good Manufacturing Practices Guidelines Drugs Used in Clinical Trials (GUI-0036).
- Guidance on Evidence to Demonstrate Drug GMP Compliance of Foreign Sites (GUI-0080) Cover Letter.
- GUIDE-0023: Risk Classification of GMP Observations, 2003 edition.
- Summary Report: Stakeholder Consultations on the Good Manufacturing Practices (GMP) Inspection Program Review (26 January 2011).
- Veterinary Drugs Annex to Current Edition of the Good Manufacturing Practices Guidelines.

3. European Union GMP Guidelines
   - EudraLex - Volume 4: Good Manufacturing Practice (GMP) Guidelines.
   - Q&A: Good Manufacturing Practice (GMP).

4. Japanese GMP Guidelines
   - GMP Compliance Inspection concerning Pharmaceuticals (including APIs).

5. US FDA GMP Guidelines
   - Center For Drug Evaluation and Research
   - Center For Veterinary Medicine
   - Center For Biologics Evaluation and Research
   - Center For Device and Radiological Health

6. World Health Organization Guidelines
   - GMP Questions and Answers.
   - Quality Assurance of Pharmaceuticals - A Compendium of Guidelines and Related Materials.

7. Australia - Therapeutic Goods Administration
   - Australian codes of good manufacturing practice - current status.

- Australian Code of Good Manufacturing Practice for Medicinal Products (16 August 2002).
- Australian Code of GMP for Human Blood and Tissues (24 August 2000).

8. Canada - Health Canada
   - Canadian Good Manufacturing Practices for Drugs (Part C Division 2 of Food and Drug Regulations).
   - Canadian GMP Resources.
9. China
   - Regulations for Implementation of the Drug Administration Law of the People's Republic of China.
10. European Union - European Medicines Agency
    - EudraLex Volume 4 - Good Manufacturing Practice Guidelines.
    - Directive 2003/94/EC for medicinal products for human use and investigational medicinal products for human use.
    - Historical Documents.
11. India - Central Drug Standard Control Organization
    - Schedule M - Good Manufacturing Practices and Requirements of Premises, Plant and Equipment For Pharmaceutical Products.
12. Japan - Pharmaceuticals and Medical Devices Agency
    - Ministerial Ordinance on Standards for Manufacturing Control and Quality Control for Drugs and Quasi-drugs (Tentative Translation VER. 09092005) [GMP] (24 December 2004).
13. United States - Food and Drug Administration GMP Regulations
    - 21 CFR Part 4 - Current Good Manufacturing Practice Requirements for Combination Products (As of 1 April 2013).
    - 21 CFR Part 210 - Current Good Manufacturing Practice in Manufacturing, Processing, Packing, or Holding of Drugs (As of 1 April 2013).

- 21 CFR Part 211 - Current Good Manufacturing Practice For Finished Pharmaceuticals- (As of 1 April 2013) Historical preambles announcing changes and comments regarding 21 CFR Parts 210 and 211.
- 21 CFR Part 212 Current Good Manufacturing Practice for Positron Emission Tomography Drugs - (As of 1 April 2013).
- 21 CFR Part 110 - Current Good Manufacturing Practice in Manufacturing, Packing, or Holding Human Food (As of 1 April 2013) Historical preambles announcing changes and comments regarding 21 CFR Part 110.
- 21 CFR Part 606 - Current Good Manufacturing Practice For Blood and Blood Components (As of 1 April 2013) Historical preambles announcing changes and comments regarding 21 CFR Part 606.
- 21 CFR Part 820 - Quality System Regulation (As of 1 April 2013).
  Historical preambles announcing changes and comments regarding 21 CFR Part 820.
- 21 CFR Part 111 - Current Good Manufacturing Practice in Manufacturing, Packaging, Labeling, or Holding Operations for Dietary Supplements (As of 1 April 2013) Historical preambles announcing changes and comments regarding 21 CFR Part 111.

14. World Health Organization
    - WHO Good Manufacturing Practices
15. Directive 2001/83/EC of the European Parliament and of the Council of 6 November 2001 on the Community code relating to medicinal products for human use. Consolidated version. December 2008.
16. Regulation (EC) No 726/2004 of the European Parliament and of the Council of 31 March 2004 laying down Community procedures for the authorization and supervision of medicinal products for human and veterinary use and establishing a European Medicines Agency. Consolidated version. July 2009.

17. Notice to applicants and regulatory guidelines medicinal products for human use. Volume 2B - Presentation and content of the dossier. Incorporating the Common Technical Document (CTD). May 2008.

18. Notice to applicants and regulatory guidelines medicinal products for human use. Volume 2A - Procedures for marketing authorization. Chapter 1 - Marketing Authorisation. November 2005.

19. Notice to applicants and regulatory guidelines medicinal products for human use. Volume 2A - Procedures for marketing authorization. Chapter 2 - Mutual Recognition. February 2007.

20. Notice to applicants and regulatory guidelines medicinal products for human use. Volume 2A - Procedures for marketing authorization. Chapter 3 - Community Referral. September 2007.

21. Notice to applicants and regulatory guidelines medicinal products for human use. Volume 2A - Procedures for marketing authorization. Chapter 4 - Centralized Procedure. April 2006.

22. Indian Pharmacopoeia

23. USP Pharmacopoeia

24. EP Pharmacopoeia

25. BP Pharmacopoeia

www.ingramcontent.com/pod-product-compliance
Lightning Source LLC
LaVergne TN
LVHW010038160826
845671LV00003B/180

* 9 7 8 9 3 8 8 3 0 5 1 4 3 *